# Multicultural Pharmaceutical Education

# Multicultural Pharmaceutical Education

Barry Bleidt, Ph.D.
Editor

Routledge
Taylor & Francis Group
New York London

First published by

**Pharmaceutical Products Press, 10 Alice Street, Binghamton, NY 13904-1580 USA.**

**Pharmaceutical Products Press is an imprint of The Haworth Press, Inc., 10 Alice Street, Binghamton, NY 13904-1580 USA.**

This edition published 2013 by Routledge

Routledge
Taylor & Francis Group
711 Third Avenue
New York, NY 10017

Routledge
Taylor & Francis Group
2 Park Square, Milton Park
Abingdon, Oxon OX14 4RN

*Routledge is an imprint of the Taylor & Francis Group, an informa business*

***Multicultural Pharmaceutical Education* has also been published as *Journal of Pharmacy Teaching*, Volume 3, Number 2 1992.**



**Library of Congress Cataloging-in-Publication Data**

**Multicultural pharmaceutical education / Barry Bleidt, editor.**
**p. cm.**
**"Has also been published as Journal of pharmacy teaching, volume 3, number 2, 1992"–T.p. verso.**
**Includes bibliographical references.**
**ISBN 1-56024-356-2 (alk. paper)** ISBN 0-7890-0071-7 (alk. paper)
**1. Pharmacy–Study and teaching–United States. 2. Afro-American pharmacists–Training of. 3. Minority pharmacists–Training of–United States. I. Bleidt, Barry.**
**[DNLM: 1. Education, Pharmacy. 2. Minority Groups–education. QV 18 M961]**
**RS110.M85 1992**
**615'.1'07173–dc20**
**DNLM/DLC**
**for Library of Congress** **92-49896**
**CIP**

# Multicultural Pharmaceutical Education

## CONTENTS

## CONCLUSION

## ABOUT THE EDITOR

**Barry A. Bleidt, Ph.D., R.Ph.,** received his B.S. Pharmacy from the University of Kentucky and his Ph.D. in Pharmacy Health Care Administration from the University of Florida. He started his academic career at Northeastern University College of Pharmacy and Allied Health Professions, Boston in 1983. He accepted a position at the University of Houston College of Pharmacy in 1987 and transferred to his current position as Associate Professor of Pharmacy Administration at Xavier University of Louisiana College of Pharmacy in 1989. Dr. Bleidt has published over thirty articles in professional and academic journals and has given over sixty presentations on management-related and other pharmaceutical topics. He has served as guest editor for the *Journal of Pharmaceutical Marketing and Management* and the *Journal of Pharmacy Teaching* and currently serves on the editorial board of *The Journal of Pharmacy Teaching* and *Clinical Research and Regulatory Affairs*. He was a Contributing Editor to *U.S. Pharmacist* and authored a column on Geriatric Pharmacy. Dr. Bleidt was the project director and host of the American Pharmaceutical Association's William S. Apple Program in Community Pharmacy Management. In addition to administering this program, he designed the curriculum and group dynamics portions of it. Dr. Bleidt is an active member of the following professional organizations: American Pharmaceutical Association, Louisiana Pharmacists Association, American Association of Colleges of Pharmacy, American Public Health Association, American Institute of the History of Pharmacy, American Society of Pharmacy Law, Southeast Louisiana Society of Hospital Pharmacists and the National Eagle Scout Association. Currently he is serving as the Program Chair for the APHA Alcohol, Tobacco and Other Drugs Section.

We have a moral and ethical responsibility to make sure that none of our African-American graduates *will ever* be in a situation where the lack of a Pharm.D. would prevent them from realizing *any* career opportunities that they desire.

*-Marcellus Grace*

# *INTRODUCTION*

## Multicultural Pharmaceutical Education: An Introduction

Barry Bleidt

The interest in increasing the number of minorities practicing pharmacy has waxed and waned over the years. Sometimes the expanded focus is due to a genuine concern for the underrepresented groups, especially when it comes to providing health care for them (historically, minorities practice more often in settings near neighborhoods or localities largely populated by their own kind). Other times this interest is temporary and NO real commitment is actually made toward alleviating the shortage of practicing minorities.

### *INTRODUCTION*

The spotlight is once again shining upon the minority representation in pharmacy issue. At the 138th Annual Meeting of the American Pharmaceutical Association, the House of Delegates passed a resolution supporting "a vigorous, long-term program for the recruitment of minority students into the pharmacy profession" (1). Their action was a reenact-

Barry Bleidt, Ph.D., is Associate Professor of Pharmacy Administration at the Xavier University of Louisiana College of Pharmacy, New Orleans, LA 70125.

 

ment of a similar move over twenty years ago (2). Maybe this time, something substantial will come of this renewed commitment.

The recent activity concerning this new-found regard for increasing minority enrollments in pharmacy schools was one impetus behind this special edition dedicated to "Muticultural Pharmaceutical Education." Another stimulus was the desire of the authors and the editor to make public their knowledge, feelings and concerns within this area.

Over forty people were solicited for input into this volume, representing interests in the following groups: African-Americans; Asian-Americans; Hispanic-Americans and Native Americans. Authors were selected because of prior scholarly activity or other unique experience in this area. The contributions that arrived are predominately geared toward African Americans. This is partly due to the fact that the editor is based at a historically black university and partly due to a much higher response rate from this group.

The purpose of this special volume is to spotlight an important topic–increasing the representation of underserved or disenfranchised groups in pharmacy schools and practice settings, thereby increasing and improving the provision of pharmaceutical services offered to them. The authors offer suggestions or commentary on multicultural pharmaceutical education. Each was invited to contribute and was reviewed accordingly. The wide array of offerings is a testimony to the importance that is placed on this issue by many. It is hoped that readers will glean ideas in order to incorporate them into their institutional commitments and thereby augment their chances of succeeding. This publication was also brought forth so excuses that are traditionally made for failures in these types of endeavors cannot be used ("we did not know how," "nothing seems to work," "what can we do," etc.).

A most interesting issue was raised during the initial, manuscript-solicitation phase of this project. One of my colleagues questioned the "authenticity of concern" that a special volume devoted to "Multicultural Pharmaceutical Education," edited by a Caucasian male, raised. Lengthy and interesting discussions ensued over the propriety of such an occurrence. Great care was taken to explain how this activity was not an attempt to exploit and that the greatest benefit would be derived by those needing it (the disenfranchised groups).

If for some reason, the reader does not understand the reasons behind or if the reader would have been defensive or insulted by such questioning, then a reevaluation of your understanding of minorities may be in order (further discussion of this point appears in the last article). However, if your cultural-sensitivity radar anticipated this concern, you will probably gain a great deal from what we have presented. Obviously, the appropriateness issue was resolved and my colleague made a valuable contribution to this collection. His concern was most appreciated.

Some ideas presented here are unique and can provide an opportunity for majority institutions to improve greatly their recruitment and retention efforts geared towards minorities. Other articles give historical accounts or examples of successes that could be emulated. However, the most important aspect of this gathering of ideas is that all of these articles are together in one publication at the same time. The Haworth Press, Inc. should be lauded for its vision in presenting the concept. I speak for most authors when I say that questions can be directed to them or to myself for assistance in implementing any ideas or programs suggested herein and we welcome them.

Contributors to this special volume range from deans to undergraduates, from vice provost to executive director and from national "Teacher of the Year" to faculty member. All have had experience in some aspect of minority pharmaceutical education. Read on, enjoy and learn.

## *WHAT'S INSIDE*

The articles that were contributed have been divided into four areas–foundation, commitment, actuation and conclusion.

### *Foundation*

The foundation portion of this special volume is provided by two articles, one on the entry-level degree and one on the right to an education. They provide the infrastructure for the rest of the collection by describing fundamental points and setting the tone for what is to follow.

In the first article, Dean Marcellus Grace, from Xavier University of Louisiana, discusses many issues relevant to muticultural pharmaceutical education, most notably the degree one. He calls Xavier's progress toward an entry-level Pharm.D. "a moral obligation." During the many forums and debates addressing this all-consuming question and in a recent presentation of "so-called research" by a professional society, an overwhelming majority of the voices have ignored what he considers as important. It is not that what Dean Grace says is so profound or will solve the crisis that is so noteworthy, it is the fact that his concerns are rarely raised or even considered. It is not possible to have commitment to minority pharmaceutical education without consideration of what issues impact upon these groups. This article speaks to that end.

The second article, by Dr. Michael Montagne of Northeastern University, presents the concept of "The Right to Learn: Advantaging the Disadvantaged Student in Pharmaceutical Education." He espouses the idea that pharmacy schools should educate people rather than the traditional train-of-thought that we should prepare students for practice. The ideological difference between the two convictions is vast.

Discrimination is a human attribute; we differentiate between things regularly. However, when biases are used as the foundation for decisions (such as race, gender, age, etc.) and they have negative impacts on others, improper discrimination has occurred. Therefore, trying to have students fit the "standard pharmacist mold" or conform to one's image of who should practice lends itself to improper biases. Hence the great concern by many about the changing demographics of pharmacy students. Not all students have the same needs and abilities, but yet many more could make an excellent contribution to pharmacy if only given the chance in an environment more responsive to their needs, rather than to those of the traditional pharmacy student. Dr. Montagne's article suggests changes in the way we view pharmaceutical education in order to become more responsive to the needs of others.

### *Commitment*

The second segment, commitment, is represented by four articles. As one ages, wisdom evolves and it becomes easier to assess the level of genuineness whenever concern is voiced on minority-centered issues. One of the major points that need to be gleaned from this segment is that minorities (and others) can differentiate between true commitment and lip service.

In the first manuscript, Dr. Robert Gibson, Associate Vice Chancellor University of California San Francisco, defines the contradictory nature of commitment and gives an historical account of its elusiveness. He also points out examples of commitment and nonexamples of such dedication to principle. And finally, he says,

> I trust health care practitioners and educators concur that the opportunity and the responsibility to improve the delivery of health care rests with each of us and also recognize that *commitment* to providing access to an education in pharmacy is part of the equation in solving the problem of the double standard of health care. (3)

This statement accents why this volume was brought forth.

The next article is by a young, clinical faculty member at Xavier University, Dr. Adrian Goram. He chronicles the commitment of historically black colleges and universities and the vital role they play in producing minority pharmacists within an ethnocentric society. He also addresses the importance of clinical rotations in preparing students for practice through integration of didactic knowledge in an applied setting and through role modeling.

The third article is about dedication to principle. It is coauthored by Michael Gerald and John Cassady from Ohio State University. It discusses "Cooperative Approaches to Stimulating Minority Participation in Graduate Pharmaceutical Education."

Several other universities are attempting to implement or have established similar affiliation agreements with minority institutions. However, this program stands out as one to be emulated. It represents commitment.

The final article of this section is about preparing minority pharmacy students for international health service. It is coauthored by Dr. Rosalyn King and Jewel Bellegarde, Director and Training Coordinator, respectively, of the International Health Institute of the Charles R. Drew University of Medicine and Science. They describe the International Health Internship Program and how it has helped to expand the "pool of minority leaders who serve the underserved wherever they are encountered."

It is ironic to note that in both the University of California San Francisco and Drew University cases, commitment was unable to continue due to budgetary constraints. This just goes to show that even when dedication is present and working, decisions from higher authorities with differing agendas and priorities can alter or destroy actuation and follow-through.

### *Actuation*

After commitment has been established, a plan needs to be formulated and actuated. This next segment presents three examples of special programs that have succeeded in their mission.

The first article in this phase is authored by Dr. J.W Carmichael et al. from Xavier University. It is especially important to point out that Dr. Carmichael recently was honored as the "National Professor of the Year" by the Council for the Advancement and Support of Education (CASE) in recognition for all that he has done in advancing science education among minorities. The innovative efforts tried by these colleagues provide good examples of how to accomplish the objective of more minorities in pharmacy education–send more through the prepharmacy pipeline better prepared through alternative teaching techniques sensitive to their needs.

The second article comes from Florida A&M University. It chronicles the growth of this historically black university in the research and graduate-education arena. Dean Johnnie Early, II et al. describe how both federal and private funding provided the foundation for their rise as a major research institution (#11 among pharmacy schools in NIH funding) and as the largest producer of African-American graduate students.

The third article in this segment is "Barriers to a Career in Pharmacy: An Hispanic Perspective" by Director Carmen Aceves-Blumenthal of Southeastern University of the Health Sciences. This is one of only two manuscripts that discusses issues of relevance specific to Hispanics. While the majority of pharmacists relish in the fact that we are the most trusted professional, some groups (such as the Hispanics) are still vying for respect from their compadres. This impacts on the decision of many whether or not to pursue a pharmacy career. In this manuscript, this barrier and others to greater Hispanic participation within the profession are described.

The final article is by a minority graduate student attending a majority institution. Carolyn Brown, from the University of Florida, is currently enrolled in the Pharmacy Health Care Administration program. She writes about her experiences and expectations. For those institutions interested in attracting such students, this article describes what it takes to do it–commitment and follow-through. Her University's devotion to these endeavors has paid dividends, both to the school in terms of attracting a more diverse student population and to the minority community by producing more role models and examples of success. Read this one carefully for useful suggestions from a person who is currently experiencing it.

## *CONCLUSION*

The last segment wraps up the collection. It contains four articles, two from pharmacy students and two from faculty.

First, two articles detail how professionalism and leadership affect student growth. In one, Dr. Edward Clouse of Southeastern University of the Health Sciences, discusses leadership training programs and preparing minority populations for leadership roles. He also details the importance of recognizing and rewarding it. As Executive Director of Phi Lambda Sigma, the National Pharmacy Leadership Society, he espouses the values of developing and acknowledging pharmacy leadership in the same manner as we have traditionally recognized and rewarded pharmacy scholarship.

In the second article, the President of the Mexican American Association of Pharmacy Students (MAAPS) at the University of Texas at Austin, Leticia de la Rosa, describes how MAAPS' activities present members with multiple opportunities to work together and support each other. This network attempts not only to help themselves, but also the underserved community around them.

In the next article, Marilyn Saulsbury of Xavier University of Louisiana, highlights the advantages of being a minority student attending a minority university. The information she provides is important for majority institutions to understand before they will become successful in attracting and retaining minority students.

The concluding article, "Understanding Minority Education in Pharmacy," presents both a summary of the entire issue and several novel concepts. The author attempts to put into words what has been working at minority institutions for many decades in advancing the educational and professional needs of disenfranchised peoples and in producing the majority of African-American pharmacists.

I wish to extend my gratitude to all authors who, through their participation, exhibited commitment by adhering to extremely short deadlines and assisting in bringing forth this collaborative effort. It is our collective wish that the information contained herein will benefit those we are trying to serve. Read on and contemplate, much can be done with the tools presented. Please try to use them for all society to benefit.

## REFERENCES

1. Anon. New policies adopted by the 1991 APhA House of Delegates. Am Pharm 1991;NS31:416-7.

2. American Pharmaceutical Association House of Delegates Notebook. 138th Annual Meeting, March 1991.

# The Entry-Level Doctor of Pharmacy Degree: Implications for Minority Pharmacists

Marcellus Grace

**SUMMARY.** The purpose of this article is to give the author's views on the B.S. vs. Pharm.D. debate from the perspective of the Dean of one of the four historically Black Colleges of Pharmacy. Data seem to indicate that all colleges/schools of pharmacy offer or soon will offer the Pharm.D. degree in the near future. The rhetorical question and criticism by many in the pharmacy profession is whether or not all graduates need the Pharm.D. degree. The author concludes that they do, and the reason is they can better market themselves.

The author states that the entry-level Pharm.D. program will have a significant impact on the African Americans and other minority pharmacists. It is predicted that given current trends, there may be a decline of African American and Hispanic pharmacy students enrolled as schools convert to the entry-level Pharm.D. The author concludes that minority pharmacists, in the future, without a Pharm.D. could face racial discrimination with the lack of a Pharm.D. being used as a potential "legitimate" excuse to not hire them in key administrative, clinical or other nontraditional roles.

Marcellus Grace, Ph.D., is Dean of the Xavier University of Louisiana College of Pharmacy, New Orleans, LA 70125.

 

> African-American pharmacists could find themselves as a "double minority"–vis à vis, with a B.S. pharmacy degree and African American.

The purpose of this article is to give my views on the B.S. vs. Pharm.D. debate from the perspective of the Dean of one of the four (4) Historically Black Colleges of Pharmacy. At the outset, let me state that these are my personal views, and do not necessarily reflect the views of the entire faculty of Xavier University's College of Pharmacy, nor that of the other three Historically Black Colleges of Pharmacy. However, the faculty unanimously adopted the entry-level Pharm.D. as our only degree.

As far back as 1948, it was suggested by the Elliott Commission that colleges establish the six-year Pharm.D. degree as the entry-level degree for all pharmacists. Two years later, the University of California became the first school of Pharmacy to adopt the Pharm.D. program. The University of Southern California followed suit, and until the early 1970s these were the only two schools offering the six-year Pharm.D. degree exclusively. By 1965, all schools had moved from a four-year B.S. to a five-year B.S. degree.

Today, 63 schools offer the B.S. in Pharmacy. Twenty-three (23) schools offer the Pharm.D. as the first professional degree; at 13 of these schools the Pharm.D. is the only Professional degree. Forty (40) schools offer the Pharm.D. as a Post B.S. degree (1). Clearly, these data indicate an indisputable trend that the Pharm.D. will eventually become the sole, entry-level degree in Pharmacy.

In a statement dated September 17, 1989, the American Council on Pharmaceutical Education Board of Directors provided notice of its intention to propose revision of accreditation standards in the 1990s within the framework of a doctor of pharmacy program. On February 15, 1990, the Executive Director of ACPE, Dr. Daniel A. Nona, published the *Procedures and Schedule for the Revision of Accreditation Standards and Guidelines (Ninth Edition) years: 1990-2000*. Part of this declaration of intent contains the following statement.

> Based upon the Council's analysis and assessment of current practice developments, future practice challenges and the corresponding educational preparedness needed, the Council foresees the time when the accreditation standards will focus upon a doctor of pharmacy program as the only professional degree program evaluated and accredited. This new direction may become adopted as soon as the year 2000.(2)

With the release of this statement, the Pharm.D. vs. B.S. debate has been set off again. The two main retail pharmacy organizations wasted no time in speaking out on the entry-level Pharm.D. program.

In a December 10, 1990 National Association of Chain Drug Stores (NACDS) News Release, a summary of the analysis on the future role of the community pharmacist was presented, along with the profound effect that policies now being debated would have on the practice of pharmacy and the provision of health care services in this country. The study was conducted by SRI International and it indicated that the most likely role of the future community pharmacist would be an expansion of the current role to one of a "drug use counselor." According to this scenario, pharmacists would spend the majority of their time counseling patients on the use of prescription and over-the-counter medications and overseeing drug distribution and control. SRI further determined that the education necessary for a community pharmacist to gain the needed competencies to play an expanded role in drug use counseling should take no more than five years to complete (3).

The National Association of Retail Druggists (NARD) conducted a survey in October 1990 of nearly 2,000 of its members. The results were released on January 16, 1991 (4). A full two-thirds of survey respondents indicated that they prefer the B.S. degree or believe that schools should be able to offer both the B.S. and Pharm.D. as entry-level degrees. Sixty-two (62) percent of the respondents indicated that five years should be sufficient to earn the entry-level Professional degree with another 10 percent expressing the view that schools should continue to offer both five and six-year, entry-level degree programs (4).

## *IS THERE A NEED FOR AN ALL PHARM.D.?*

The rhetorical question and criticism by many in our profession is, do all pharmacists need a Pharm.D. degree? Dr. John Gans' answer is the best that I have heard to date. His answer, in part, is . . . "No, not in all settings. But no one can guarantee where a student is going to practice" (5). Dr. Gans goes on to make the point that today's Pharmacy B.S. graduates practicing into the year 2030 and beyond will be limited. The Pharm.D. degree will enable our graduates to market themselves better. "Then, whether a student achieves or not will be based on his or her competency, postgraduate experiences and motivation" (5). I agree wholeheartedly with this statement. The degree should not be the limiting factor in any of our graduates achieving their pharmacy career goals.

## *IMPACT ON BLACK AND OTHER MINORITY PHARMACISTS*

The entry-level Pharm.D. program will have a significant impact on African Americans and other minority pharmacists. The production of Pharm.D.'s has been going up consistently since AACP began to gather data on the degree in 1960. Since 1985, the production of entry-level Pharm.D.'s had increased an average of 18.8 percent per year (6). It is quite interesting when one does an analysis of trends of Pharm.D.'s among minority graduates. From 1976 to 1989, there were 7,258 Pharm.D.'s awarded as the first degree, of these only 274 (3.8%) were African American and 242 (3.3%) were Hispanic. From 1973 to 1989 there were 3,321 Pharm.D.'s awarded as second degrees (post B.S.), only 119 (3.6%) were African American and 51 (1.5%) were Hispanic. All total, both first and second degree Pharm.D.'s were 10,579; three hundred ninety-three (393) or 3.7 percent were African American and two hundred ninety three (293) or 2.8 percent Hispanic (6).

To do a comparison of B.S. and Pharm.D. degrees conferred on minorities, I totaled the number of B.S. degrees conferred from 1972 to 1989 which came to 110,350. Of these, 3,898 (3.5%) were African Americans and 4,405 (4%) Hispanics. It is interesting to note that the percent of B.S. and Pharm.D.'s for African Americans is exactly the same (3.5%). For Hispanics, there is a higher percentage for B.S. (4%) vs. 2.8 percent for Pharm.D.'s.

Even though there have been slight increases in enrollment among African American students since the mid-1970s, it seems as though the percentage receiving degrees, both B.S. and Pharm.D., has remained constant at around 3.5 percent. With the trend towards the entry-level Pharm.D. degree, most schools have reduced their enrollments when they converted to these programs. This might suggest that one can predict a decline proportionately of African Americans and Hispanics in our schools of pharmacy in the future.

Another troublesome fact is that even in 1988 only 4,800 pharmacists were African American (7). This is estimated to be about 3 percent of the pharmacists in active practice. While the data is unknown, my best estimate is that only approximately 450 of these pharmacists (9.4%) hold Pharm.D. degrees. The trend is quite disturbing when you consider that in 1950 only 1.4 percent of the pharmacists were African American, in 1980 this increased to 2.3 percent (8). So in a period of over 40 years we've only been able to increase the number of African American Pharmacists by only 1.6 percent.

Already, many positions such as clinical coordinators, directors of hospital pharmacies, clinical trial monitoring, etc., require a Pharm.D. degree. While one does not hear of any flagrant or overt discrimination against the hiring and promotion of African-American pharmacists, the lack of a Pharm.D. could, in fact, be used as a potential "legitimate" excuse not to hire African-American pharmacists for certain key administrative, "clinical" or other nontraditional pharmacist practitioner roles. If one is not careful, African-American pharmacists could conceivably find themselves as a "double minority"–vis à vis with a B.S. pharmacy degree and African-American. Think ahead to the year 2030 or so and a significant number of African-American pharmacists could be relegated to the lower level B.S. dispensing pharmacy jobs while many other higher level and diverse practice settings and career opportunities could potentially be denied to them because of the lack of a Pharm.D. degree.

## *WHAT HAS XAVIER UNIVERSITY DONE TO ADDRESS THIS ISSUE?*

In the spring of 1986, Xavier University's Board of Trustees approved the implementation of a twenty-three (23) month post-baccalaureate Doctor of Pharmacy program. We took four students in the fall of 1987, and in May, 1990, we graduated our first class of four students. Recognizing the impending movement to an all Pharm.D. program by the year 2000, I charged the faculty in the Fall of 1989 to develop a six-year, entry-level program and revise the 23-month, post-baccalaureate program to a 13-month program. In the spring of 1990, a final curriculum was overwhelmingly approved by the Xavier faculty.

Therefore, beginning in the Fall of 1991, Xavier will admit its first, entry-level Pharm.D. class. The revised, 13-month, post-B.S. Pharm.D. program will also begin then. The last B.S. class was admitted in the Fall of 1990; these students are expected to complete their degrees by May 1993. The first all Pharm.D. class should graduate in May 1995. In 1994, there will be a B.S. class of all students who were unable, for various reasons to complete their curriculum by 1993. However, I should hasten to add that all students who entered in the last B.S. class were told by a formal letter and verbally when they enrolled, that B.S. course offering availability beyond the Spring of 1993 would be very limited.

At Xavier, we have projected budgets over the next five to six years to phase in the entry-level program. The greatest impact will be the need to add approximately seven FTE, clinical faculty to cover the additional year of clerkships.

One major argument presented by the opponents of the all Pharm.D. degree is that it will have an adverse effect on an already short supply of pharmacists. In Xavier's case, it is true that the class of 1994 will be a relatively small class, but we expect to admit at least 100 students or more in the Fall of 1991, and we just admitted 100 students in the last B.S. class. We are projecting a graduating class for 1991 of approximately 109 students. Therefore, we feel that we will actually be able to increase our class sizes rather than decrease them. It is important to note that this Fall, Xavier experienced a 13% enrollment increase from last Fall to a record breaking total of 341 pharmacy students and some 300 in prepharmacy.

Our enrollment success can be attributed to having two full-time recruiters with adequate travel funding to do targeted national recruiting. Xavier is still the number one ranked pharmacy school in the country, in terms of enrolling some fifteen percent of all African-Americans studying pharmacy. We have also produced approximately twenty-five percent of the 4,800 African-American pharmacists in practice today.

While we feel at Xavier our enrollments will increase with increased recruiting efforts, this enthusiasm has to be tempered with the realization of some negative factors. The first major concern overall is the drop in African-American youth who are entering college. In 1976, almost 33 percent of African American and white youth who graduated from high school moved on to college. By 1987, the rate increased to 37 percent for whites but fell to 29 percent among African Americans (9). The second major factor facing future minority pharmacy students will be their ability to finance their education. At Xavier, some 85-90 percent of our students receive some form of financial aid. The debt burden continues to increase each year, as tuition and related cost rise; the amount of financial assistance continues to diminish and is shifting more and more towards loans. Many Xavier pharmacy students are graduating currently with loans which average $32-35,000. The cost for the one additional year could discourage some students from entering pharmacy programs.

In spite of these potential obstacles to our future students, it is my personal opinion that a minority college of pharmacy like Xavier can ill afford to run the risk of producing a "soon to be obsolete degree." In spite of the current debate, I feel that the entry-level Pharm.D. is eventually going to happen. Therefore, I feel that my faculty and I have made the correct decision to move forward with the entry-level degree. As such Xavier will be able to continue its 64-year history of graduating well-trained pharmacists who will be prepared to practice pharmacy in the year 2030 and beyond.

## *CONCLUSION*

In conclusion, Xavier University's College of Pharmacy has taken the challenge to prepare African American pharmacists for the future at the all Pharm.D. level and feels prepared to continue our 64-year history of distinguished pharmacy education.

For the practitioners who want to upgrade their B.S. credentials to our Pharm.D. level, the post-baccalaureate, 13-month program will offer part-time courses, television courses, future plans for home study, and potential academic credit for previous experiences.

*We also have a moral and ethical responsibility to make sure that none of our African American graduates* will ever *be in a situation where the lack of a Pharm.D. would prevent them from realizing* any *career opportunities that they desire.*

## REFERENCES

1. American Association of Colleges of Pharmacy. Vital statistics–program in pharmacy. Alexandria, VA: American Association of Colleges of Pharmacy, August 1990.

2. Nona DA. Procedures and schedule for the revision of accreditation standards and guidelines (ninth edition) years: 1990-2000. Chicago: ACPE, 15 February 1990.

3. Anon. An assessment of future educational needs for community pharmacists. Final report. SRI International, SRI project 1057, December, 1990.

4. Anon. NARD news release. 16 January 1991.

5. Gans JA. Freedom of opportunity: the Pharm.D. degree. Am Pharm 1990;NS30:328-31.

6. Penna RP, Sherman MS. Degrees conferred by schools and colleges of pharmacy 1988-89. Alexandria, VA: American Association of Colleges of Pharmacy.

7. Seventh report to the President and Congress on the status of health personnel in the United States. DHS Publication No. HRS-P-OD-90-1. March 1990.

8. Hauft RS, Fishman LE, Evans WJ. Blacks and the health professions in the 80's: a national crisis and a time for action. Association of Minority Health Professions Schools, June 1983.

9. Anon. Trends in the post secondary enrollment of minorities. RAND Corporation, 13 November 1990.

# The Right to Learn: Advantaging the Disadvantaged Student in Pharmaceutical Education

Michael Montagne

**SUMMARY.** The concept that any person, who wishes to assume the role of being a student, has a right to learning opportunities is presented and discussed. Disadvantageous situations involving students occur regularly in pharmaceutical education. Proactive policies and procedures need to be developed and implemented to provide advantages in those instances where students already are placed at a disadvantage. Providing ethical and cross-cultural experiences in the curriculum, and in the educational institution as a whole, are imperative. Even more important, our values and beliefs regarding the interrelated, yet distinct, notions of higher education, professional licensure, and occupational employment need to be clarified and understood by those involved in the educational process.

Unless a student is a white, male person of Western European heritage (and American-born) without any disabilities or infirmities, he or she more than likely will face prejudice, bias, and a variety of barriers in their pursuit of a pharmaceutical education. Many educators and practitioners wrongly unite the learning of pharmaceutical knowledge with a specific job in pharmaceutical practice. This, in addition to ethnocentric beliefs and misperceptions about individuals who do not fit the social or professional norm (as represented by the dominant person-type), leads to greater disadvantages for the already disadvantaged student.

This author argues that, in principle, every person has the *right* to a

Michael Montagne, Ph.D., is Associate Professor of Social Pharmacy at the Northeastern University College of Pharmacy and Allied Health Professions, 113 Mugar Hall, 360 Huntington Ave., Boston, MA 02115.

 

pharmaceutical education, regardless of genetic, physiological, psychological, social, intellectual, or moral deficiencies. The issue of whether a person should be licensed to practice pharmacy, or whether he or she should hold a specific job or position in the pharmaceutical profession, is separate and distinct from their right to learn. Providing opportunities to learn must be free of these latter biases. A better understanding of the relationship between education, professional acceptance and licensure, and specific occupational placement is needed to prevent further barriers to learning about drugs, pharmacy, and the pharmaceutical sciences (1). First, some real life examples may be instructive to this argument.

## *PREJUDICE AND ETHNOCENTRISM IN PHARMACY: FOUR CASES FROM MY CAREER*

At my current university, educational opportunities for the hearing impaired are promoted, and as a result, a few students have chosen pharmacy as a career path. While the response by faculty here has been positive and supportive, faculty at other schools and many practitioners have expressed doubts and concerns. The true problematic nature of those beliefs confronted me when a former girlfriend, who is a pharmacist, chastised me for allowing such students to matriculate, stating that "they should not be allowed in pharmacy school" with the argument "how could they possibly practice in a pharmacy?" If we dissuade hearing impaired people from having an opportunity to study the pharmaceutical sciences, let alone practice in a specific pharmacy setting (which really is not a decision for an educator to make), would we stop there, or would we include the visually impaired, chemically impaired, and others? By the way, these hearing impaired graduates are currently licensed and practicing in very traditional settings that are conducive to and supportive of their abilities.

At an institution where I previously taught, I was asked to be the nonclinical member of the Pharm.D. Admissions Committee. At the first meeting, file folders for each applicant were passed around. The procedure for selecting candidates for a campus interview was described; they were chosen based upon "good looks" (a color photograph was required in the application materials and it was prominently displayed on the *outside* of the folder), and racial and gender characteristics were major considerations. Applicants were invited for an interview based upon the criterion of "what a clinical pharmacist should look like." One candidate, who appeared "very white" in her photograph, was instead of

African-American heritage, much to the consternation of some committee members. While I did voice my objection to this procedure, and tried to delineate both its illogical and biased aspects, to my shame I did not say anything to the Dean nor resign in protest from the committee. It is a lesson I carry with me to this day.

At some institutions, I have noticed that pharmacists, who are clerkship and externship preceptors, treat certain patients (with AIDS, cancer, sexually-transmitted and other diseases) in uncaring, unsupportive, inattentive and other biased ways. This was not new nor surprising to me, but what was new is the extension of these behaviors to students with the same conditions, with the belief that people with such illnesses "should not be let into the pharmacy profession." How far do we go with this way of thinking? Those people with AIDS, cancer, epilepsy, psychiatric disorders, perhaps even homosexuality, and who knows what else, need not apply to our school nor seek careers in our profession! I call this the "Epidemic of Unfeeling Pharmaceutical Professionals."

Throughout my career, I have observed that different, and usually more difficult, standards for admission to, passing courses in, and graduation from pharmacy schools apply to international students. This consists of "extra" assignments or criteria in "jumping through the hoops" on the way to a degree in pharmacy. This also includes requiring an extensive and complete re-education for those with pharmaceutical degrees, licensure, and even years of practice in pharmacy in another country. On the other hand, if they, their parents, or governments have enough money, they seem to have little problem in gaining admittance into some pharmacy schools. I call this the "American Pharmacy is the *Only* Quality Pharmacy and All Foreign Education and Practice are Second Rate" Syndrome.

## *THE DISADVANTAGING OF STUDENTS IN PHARMACEUTICAL EDUCATION*

Whether he or she is a student or practicing pharmacist, a patient, a scientist or teacher, a faculty member or administrator, you cannot look only at one part of that person; you must view that person as a whole. There are distinctions between education (and the right to learn) and being a health professional (and the privilege of practicing pharmacy). It is my philosophy that education is the process of teaching, guiding, engaging a person's mind in his or her pursuit of personal development. It is the act of providing an opportunity to learn. Professional licensure, on the other hand, is the process of determining who should be registered (allowed) to practice in that profession, whether or not they actually choose to do so. Job placement, or employment, is the occupational activity of deciding who fulfills certain job requirements, and who specifically should assume a given position in an organizational (work place) hierarchy. There is a great need for compassion, for understanding the differences between, and for a rational approach to educating, licensing, and employing student and practicing pharmacists.

Virtually all colleges and universities have pledged to provide all of their students with a nondiscriminatory academic environment, free of intimidation, coercion, and unfair treatment based on race, religion, ethnic or national origin, age, gender, handicap, or veteran status, and in some cases sexual preference. This goal applies to all matters involving admissions and registration, and in all official relationships with students, including evaluation of academic performance. Most policies of this type also condemn sexual harassment.

The latest enrollment data for schools and colleges of pharmacy (1989-90) show that Asian Americans represent 9.2%, Black Americans represent 6.7%, and Hispanic Americans represent 3.7% of all students enrolled for an entry level degree (2). Students of Native American descent and other foreign-born students are much smaller in number. From 1985, Asian American enrollment has increased 92%, Black American enrollment has increased 19%, and Hispanic American enrollment has increased 18% (2). While the number of foreign-born students enrolled in graduate programs is great, the proportion of those from American-born minority groups is abysmally small. Representation of minority groups amongst pharmaceutical faculty also is embarrassingly small. Do these results indicate progress, and if so, to what degree?

State pharmacy board requirements for sitting for licensure examination include age (18 in most states), U.S. citizenship, graduation from an accredited school or college of pharmacy, and a certain minimum number of internship (practical experience) hours. The awarding of licensure to practice pharmacy consists solely of showing a minimum competency (i.e., passing the examination), and of not having broken the law (e.g., conviction of a felony offense). State boards also indicate that applications for licensure and examinations will be reviewed in a nondiscriminatory manner. It has been noted, however, that there is a legal monopoly inherent in professional licensing (3). In addition, the pharmaceutical curriculum at many schools is designed more for passing the state board examination, than for a foundation of knowledge in the pharmaceutical sciences. Most state boards also say that a pharmacy shall not limit its services to a particular segment or segments of the general public.

One recent well-known example of prejudice in health care delivery is refusing treatment of HIV-positive patients, which is a violation of professional and ethical standards, and should not be tolerated (4). In a recent commentary, a pharmacist described what happened upon learning that he is HIV-positive: "If it helps pharmacists to read about HIV infection without prejudice because I am neither homosexual nor an i.v. drug abuser, I am willing to go public" (4). His employers are very supportive of his continuing to work, though other people in his life may be less so. But in reflecting upon his quote, the reason for publishing his story, I think how unfortunate it must be for those HIV-positive pharmacists who instead have a certain sexual preference or route of administration in their drug taking.

Employment usually is considered as being "at will" (5). But now there are statutory exceptions to this doctrine precluding unjustified dismissal in areas involving civil rights, labor unions, workman's compensation, health and safety, refusal to take a polygraph (and in some cases, drug testing), and of course, refusing to violate public law, regulations, or policy, or to engage in unprofessional conduct (5).

Distinctions are made in employment between discrimination and bias. Selecting employees (in our case, students) should involve a process in which some individuals are discriminated from others and thus selected or rejected (6). If a process or system does not elicit variability among candidates, then it does not provide useful information to distinguish or differentiate and thus to make a decision, when given limited resources. What is crucial is whether the discriminations are fair or free of bias. What is fair or biased also can be difficult to determine. A key principle of one basic employment approach is instructive: "unfair discrimination or bias is said to exist when members of a minority group have lower probabilities of being selected for a job when, in fact, if they had been selected, their probabilities of performing successfully would have been equal to those of nonminority group members" (6). The Federal Government takes the approach that a selection process which has an adverse impact is discriminatory (7).

What does all of this have to do with a distinction between education and practice? I have a license to practice pharmacy, but I have not done so for 10 years. It would be ludicrous for me to engage in any aspect of distributive, managerial, or clinical pharmacy without significant retraining. Yet my license allows me to apply immediately for a position in most any type of pharmacy practice setting. It is the responsibility of the employer to reject my application, to suggest retraining, or to accept me under direct supervision of someone more experienced. So should certain individuals, on the other hand, be prevented from practicing pharmacy for any reason, and what specifically are those reasons?

## PROVIDING ADVANTAGES AND THE RIGHT TO LEARN

American society, distinct from most others, supports and provides many freedoms for the individual over the society that wants to dominate them. It is evident in the expression of ethical principles such as autonomy and of political stances such as libertarianism. How do we allow these values to grow and flourish in an educational setting? We provide unbiased opportunities to learn.

The principle most widely used in mission statements of pharmacy schools is "preparation of students for practice" (8). Other principles, or goals if you will, include: the preparation of students for advanced professional or graduate education; to become responsible health professionals; for participation on health care teams; and even to instill loyalty to their institutions. Only one principle mentioned in some of these statements had any focus on learning as a component of their mission. It is "to prepare graduates for lifelong learning." Further categorical analysis of those mission statements found that only 13% of the schools indicated that they attempted "to maintain an environment for learning" and only 2% indicated that they tried "to provide for scholarly development" (8).

AACP's new mission statement for pharmaceutical education states "pharmaceutical education is responsible for preparing students to enter into the practice of pharmacy and to function as professionals and informed citizens in a changing health care system." In recent publications, it has been noted that "our obligation as educators and as pharmacists is to provide society with the mix of professionals that it needs, wants, and can afford" (9). The argument by many is that we in pharmaceutical education should identify and educate those people who potentially are most suitable for practice. But should we be the screening agent and perform *de facto* differentiation of those who could versus those who could not pass a state board examination, obtain a license, or be most marketable to employers or most valuable to society? How often have we in educational institutions heard remarks, or even seen decisions being made, based upon these beliefs?

As Robert Hutchins, the great innovative president of the University of Chicago in the 1930s and 1940s, remarked "professional education consists either of going through motions that we have inherited or of making gestures of varying degrees of wildness that we hope may be more effectual" (10). The problem, he felt, was a love of money that besets universities, private or public. "The universities are dependent on the people. The people love money and think that education is a way of getting it. They think too that democracy means that every child should be permitted to acquire the educational insignia that will be helpful in making money. They do not believe in the cultivation of the intellect for its own sake" (10). The conflict then is between two kinds of education, the pursuit of knowledge (or learning) for its own sake and the preparation of people for their work or careers.

Plato embodied the principle of equal educational opportunity in *The Republic*, and Jefferson put it into his 1779 Bill for the More General Diffusion of Knowledge. Justice Earl Warren in 1954 stated: "It is doubtful that any person may reasonably be expected to succeed in life if he is denied the opportunity of an education. Such an opportunity is a *right* which must be made available on equal terms" (11). The child's right to education received emphasis in the International Year of the Child, 1979, along with the right to nutrition, love, medical care, a name and nationality (12). The condition for something to be a human right is that it is necessary to enable the person to become a human being to the best of his or her potential, in order to sustain them in the society in which they live.

## *CHANGES FOR ALL OF US IN PHARMACEUTICAL EDUCATION*

What does disenfranchisement do to self-image, aspiration, and achievement? What is being reflected in our use of terms such as "educationally disadvantaged," "academically underprepared," "learning disabled or deficient," or even "minority?" Prejudice does prevent or limit human growth, and it is the reason for many other societal problems (13). To say that prejudice occurs in other professions and occupations, in education, or in many parts of everyday life is not an excuse. There is a big difference between legislative or regulatory reactions and social or moral responses to this problem. In other words, Equal Opportunity Employment and Affirmative Action programs in educational settings do not guarantee that prejudice will cease to exist and influence students' lives (14).

As individuals, we need to look inside ourselves, and we must identify and contemplate our own beliefs and behaviors. Both faculty and students (and even practitioners who are part of the educational process) need to promote genuine coherent pluralism throughout the campus and in all phases of the curriculum (15,16). There also is a need to ensure flexibility in the otherwise rigid use of only quantifiable admission criteria in the student selection process (11). These notions of equity and fairness should extend to all aspects of a student's life while in school.

In education, in general, we need to allow both students and faculty to gain experiences in examining ethical dilemmas, developing professional behaviors, and clarifying values (3). Specific programs should be instituted, faculty trained, curricula modified, and extracurricular or professional activities developed to fulfill these goals. At some institutions, a greater cultural awareness is achieved through intercultural communication course work, the application of cross-cultural principles to health and illness, support and encouragement of American-born minority and international students, the development of sister-school relationships (especially with schools in developing or politically-oppressed countries), and even in the renewed interest in bilingual programs and activities (17-23). What did we lose when we deleted a language requirement from the curriculum? It is time perhaps to reconsider such a requirement.

I believe that societies should devote their obviously limited resources and time to human development, and thus education (and of course, nutrition, shelter, and general well-being) than to wars, complete development of the global landmass, minor alterations in products (including pharmaceuticals) and services, or activities and enterprises that result primarily in monetary or material gains rather than knowledge, understanding, and the resolution of human problems. How important does it become in education, when people are not being paid, but instead are paying, for a service (course work)? They should not be required solely to complete a task, such as earn a degree (get that piece of parchment), but instead they should work at fulfilling goals at different rates based more upon their own motivations, time, and sense of involvement. This addresses the whole issue of a society providing resources for all or only a portion of its members to become educated. Should every human being have the right to learn, and thus at the very least, should everyone who so desires be offered the opportunity to obtain an education (14)? This will rest not on laws and regulations, nor on policies and procedures, but on our values, attitudes, and behaviors toward one another in every aspect of our daily lives.

## REFERENCES

1. Vogt DD, Montagne M, Smith HA. Science and technology in American pharmacy practice education. Am J Pharm Educ 1981;45:232-7.

2. Penna RP, Sherman MS. Enrollments in schools and colleges of pharmacy, 1989-1990. Am J Pharm Educ 1990;54:451-77.

3. Myers MJ, Montagne M. Ethics. In: Gennaro AR, ed. Remington's pharmaceutical sciences. 18th ed. Easton, PA: Mack Publishing, 1990:20-7.

4. Huffman MD. On being an HIV-positive pharmacist. Am J Hosp Pharm 1991;48:148-50.

5. Simonsmeier LM. Topical update on: legal issues surrounding the pharmacist's duty to counsel patients, employment law and mail-order pharmacy. Am J Pharm Educ 1989;53:73-7.

6. Arvey RD. Fairness in selecting employees. Reading, MA: Addison-Wesley Publishing Co., 1979.

7. Adoption by four agencies of uniform guidelines on employee selection procedures (1978). Fed Register 43(25 Aug 1978):38295-309.

8. Smith MC. An analysis of pharmacy education mission statements. Am J Pharm Educ 1987;51:144-7.

9. Levy G. The Pharm.D.: all or some? DICP Ann Pharmacother 1991;25:94-7.

10. Hutchins RM. The higher learning in America. New Haven, CT: Yale University Press, 1936.

11. American Association of State Colleges and Universities. Minorities in public higher education: at a turning point. Washington, DC: AASCU Press, 1988.

12. Vandenberg D. Human rights in education. New York: Philosophical Library, 1983.

13. Allport GW. The nature of prejudice. Garden City, NY: Doubleday, 1958.

14. Weinberg M. A chance to learn: the history of race and education in the United States. New York: Cambridge University Press, 1977.

15. LeVine RA, Campbell DT. Ethnocentrism: theories of conflict, ethnic attitudes, and group behavior. New York: Wiley, 1972.

16. Musgrove F. Education and anthropology: other cultures and the teacher. New York: John Wiley and Sons, 1982.

17. Gudykunst WB. Culture and interpersonal communication. Newbury Park, CA: Sage, 1988.

18. Hall ET. Beyond culture. Garden City, NY: Anchor Press, 1976.

19. Boulding E. Building a global civic culture: education for an interdependent world. New York: Teachers College Press, 1988.

20. Kilwein JH. Science, the human condition and pharmacy. Pharm Int 1982;12:202-4.

21. Kilwein JH. Cross-cultural perspectives of health and illness: an elective course. Am J Pharm Educ 1985;49:274-6.

22. Appelt GD. Intercultural drug use: an elective course in the pharmacy curriculum. Am J Pharm Educ 1984;48:275-7.

23. Montagne M, Tarasevicius ET, Kulunis R, Bleidt BA. Pharmacy in Lithuania and the development of a sister-school relationship between colleges of pharmacy. Am J Hosp Pharm 1991;48:1035-8.

# The Commitment to Minority Recruitment Programs

Robert D. Gibson

**SUMMARY.** A myriad of programs have been mounted to increase access for the underrepresented into health career programs, some being more successful than others. Commitment is the theme of this paper and is linked to success through discussions of: the background to the health care problem in which race, income and related socioeconomic variables play dominant roles; the issue of minority access to college; the minority manpower shortages/maldistribution controversy; and, the need to secure and commit financial resources which, as an expression for diversity, would lead to the improvement of the delivery of pharmaceutical care for all the citizens of this country.

WE THE PEOPLE . . . with these words the Preamble to the Constitution of the United States eloquently set forth a new national ethos designed to guide a fledgling political experiment.

That unity of purpose, dedication to principle, and commitment to equal opportunity and progress which were to characterize the American

Robert D. Gibson, Pharm.D., is Associate Vice Chancellor for Student Academic Affairs at the University of California-San Francisco, 500 Parnassus Ave., MU200, San Francisco, CA 94015.

 

people often seems elusive and contradictory. In its stead we too frequently see an increase in the polarization and fracturing of our society, where angry individuals are pitted against each other on all fronts . . . social, economic, and political. And the phenomena is as evident in health professions education as it is in most other examples to be placed before an audience as sophisticated as pharmacy educators and practitioners.

Although the *Constitution* may guarantee that all men are created equal, it does not assure that they are treated equally. It seems to me that one of the reasons for this is that our society embraces the Horatio Alger ethic that those who truly and sincerely want to make it in our society most assuredly will. According to this formula, the poor, the uneducated, the disabled, the ill, and the unsuccessful are that way because they choose to be. It follows, therefore, that social deprivation, bad housing, malnutrition, and a host of other adversities, are not societal priorities because these conditions are self-inflicted by those who are poor, uneducated, disabled, ill, and unsuccessful. Unfortunately, the compassion of this administration for overcoming these conditions rates somewhere between its affection for Saddam Hussein and its affection for your average welfare mother, and is a nonexample of commitment.

Unlike machines and computers, the society of man is riddled with contradiction, inconsistency and conflict. For example, at a time when many scientists are striving to increase the quality and span of life, others are devising more efficient ways of taking lives, scorching the earth, and polluting the environment. The tragedy is that the contradictions, inconsistencies, and conflicts are all so unnecessary. Life is so dear and the quality of life so inexpensive that our society should be able to provide access to self-improvement for those who want to achieve. But it has not and will not for as long as it refuses to cope with the changes that have taken place and the changes that will continue to occur at an ever-accelerating pace. For example, tomorrow's world will be crowded and ways will have to be found to cope with the masses. Shifting demographics, increasing numbers of the elderly and the minorities, for example, will have a profound impact on society at large. Its priorities will shift and its democratic voice will increasingly respond to the demands of the elderly and the new majority of today's minorities. Our challenge is to persuade our institutions, whether public or private, and their decision makers, and all the other segments of society as well, to address all of the issues relevant to health professions education. We must make certain that access to a health professions education and the delivery of health care services is available to all segments of our society to ensure that the present double standard of health care will disappear.

## *BACKGROUND: ACCESS TO HEALTH CARE AND HEALTH PROFESSIONS EDUCATION*

Some twenty years ago, November 19, 1971, The Honorable William R. Roy, U.S. House of Representatives stated during a hearing before the Committee on Ways and Means, House of Representatives, 92nd Congress on National Health Insurance Proposals, "*There is no area of human life more important to an individual than his health, and there can be no area of policy of greater importance to a nation than the health of all of its people*"(1). That statement recognized, regardless of status and position, access to health care is a constitutionally guaranteed inalienable right and that members of the health professions are expected to render health services of acceptable quality to underprivileged patients as well as to advantaged persons.

That the broad diversity of the population of this country is not adequately represented in those who graduate from high school, and fewer of those are academically eligible for entrance into college, has been the focus of educators for many years. We in pharmacy education know that many of the reasons for low minority enrollment in health professions schools include inadequate preprofessional preparation, high educational costs combined with limited financial aid, cultural barriers, lack of role models, and motivation. It is also apparent that many communities in our nation are comprised of persons who, for economic, social, and cultural reasons have not enjoyed the normal privileges, rights, and opportunities inherent in an affluent society. Regardless of status and position, however, the Constitution guarantees certain inalienable rights, and access to health care is one of those rights. Yet, health statistics of the minorities and the poor confirm that the delivery of health services of acceptable quality and quantity has not been delivered to the underprivileged.

Studies made in the 1960s and 70s concluded that there was either a shortage or maldistribution of health care personnel, thereby creating a problem with access to quality health care. These academic exercises are necessary and deeply immerse us in the evolution of change, but they provide little comfort or relief for the poor, hungry, malnourished, crippled and diseased. Other studies identified that approximately one-fourth of those within this nation's social fabric of poor, hungry and malnourished were the ethnically and culturally different socioeconomically disadvantaged.

I believe it is safe to say that during the era being described Americans were shocked to learn that approximately one-fourth of the nation's population was poor. The poor had become an invisible group (if they were white) whose poverty was hidden beneath their apparent similarity to other Americans. They appeared to be healthy, they betrayed few of the signs of despair and desperation that characterize the poor in other parts of the world, and they wore much the same clothes as do we of the nonpoor classification. And, unless they were easily identified as *minorities* they were alluded to as "The other America."

But black, brown, red and yellow America was something else. It was there; everyone knew it, but it had become a phantom population in public housing, segregated middle-class neighborhoods, migrant farm workers housing, federally supported reservation domiciles or remote marginal farms in the deep south. However, as a result of the 1950s and 60s civil rights movement the poor were no longer invisible. They constituted a revolutionary force in American society for their condition was inextricably woven with other than economic issues, such as civil rights, civil dissent and the morality of war. Thus, it was no longer possible to deal with the poor solely in terms of living standards. (Author's note: Because of the economic progress minorities have made since the civil rights activities of the 1960s, it may be difficult for the reader to envision that prior to the civil rights movement a major segment of the minority population fit into the economic definition of poor.)

Eliot L. Richardson, then Secretary, Department of Health, Education, and Welfare, in a presentation on The National Health Insurance Partnership Act before the House Committee on Ways and Means (October 19, 1971) stated that lower income groups and racial minorities have far poorer health, but at the same time receive far less health service than other groups. Those gross measures masked large disparities in health status among subpopulations in the U.S. On nearly every index, the poor and the racial minorities fared worse than their opposites, e.g., shorter life spans; more chronic and debilitating illnesses; higher infant and maternal death rate, etc. (2). And, they also had far less access to health services.

Accordingly, it was recognized that awareness of these differences among our citizens . . . the denial to some of a life span as long and as relatively free of disabilities and illnesses as that which others enjoy . . . accompanied by a sense of injustices that denial entails, and by experiences that denial and its effects can and should be obviated, would be a major step in eliminating what was then known as a "health care crisis."

The above was generally accepted as an adequate description of part of the health care problem in which race, income and related socioeconomic variables played dominant roles. What followed was the consideration of the variables to eliminate this problem. The result was an agreement that reforms in education, which meant access to an education in pharmacy in particular, was to be embraced. This meant that changes in basic commitments and attitudes, as well as the commitment of financial resources to assist the poor in obtaining an education in pharmacy, were necessary and must be made available.

## *MINORITY ACCESS TO HIGHER EDUCATION/PHARMACEUTICAL EDUCATION*

The issue of minority access to college was one of the dominant issues of the 1970s and, 20 years later, still is. Around that issue revolved a host of questions and problems related to the gravity of racial and ethnic conflicts, and the answers to delivery of health care to those not receiving is partially tied, if not significantly interwoven, into *access* to higher education. Access for the poor is mostly economically controlled. Lack of ability, for example, is not a barrier to entry into the first grade of elementary school, but it is at the point of entry to college. If society were to decide that everyone must go to college, just as it decided years ago that all must attend elementary school, the ability barrier would disappear because it would be irrelevant.

The same observation could be made about barriers caused by lack of money. If it were to be decided that all the direct and indirect costs of higher education were to be charged against society at large and that the individual consumer of education would be charged nothing, the cost barrier would disappear. The point is that barriers came into being and now continue to operate because society either permitted them to evolve or consciously created them.

Some 55 years have elapsed since Lee and Jones first concluded that there was a shortage of physicians in the United States (3). Those conclusions were then extrapolated to indicate that there may also be a *shortage of pharmacists*. Thus, on the basis of more refined data, and prognostications somewhat less refined, it became fashionable to blame the insufficiencies of the health care delivery system on maldistribution. Those academic exercises were necessary, and deeply immersed us in the evolution of change, but they provided little comfort or relief for the poor, hungry, malnourished, crippled and diseased. For these were (are) the victims of either *professional manpower shortages* and/or *maldistribution*.

With respect to commitment, the attitudes of professional practitioners, and the lack of leadership from local, state, and national pharmaceutical associations cannot escape indictment. The past had demonstrated that all of the above have, to differing degrees, either neglected or refused to initiate without prodding any activity to increase minority enrollment in pharmacy schools. Back in 1971, during the annual meeting of the American Pharmaceutical Association, the association was sharply criticized by members of its House of Delegates for not delivering on its policy, adopted a year earlier, to make special efforts to recruit disadvantaged ethnic and racial minorities. The point is that the challenge to assist in increasing the number of health professionals from minority groups was accepted only after a confrontation over priorities. Unfortunately, the priorities were related to minority recruitment specifically rather than to improvement in the delivery of pharmaceutical services generally through minority recruitment. By and large, local and state associations made the same kinds of noises but not the commitments necessary to move ahead with minority recruitment.

## *MINORITY MANPOWER ARGUMENT AND COMMITMENT*

To recite forecasts and provide documentation which indicates that pharmacy manpower demands will exceed the supply and to use these forecasts as a basis for committing ourselves to minority recruitment is specious reasoning. It enshrouds the real issue. To design recruitment strategy on the premise that pharmacy manpower requirements dictate tapping of the potential minority manpower is not facing, or refusing to recognize, the real issue of socioeconomic discrimination, whether de facto or otherwise. It is a cop out.

The determination of whether or not to commit ourselves makes the difference between a paper plan to be filed and a commitment to a viable entity. Commitment is the most important aspect to be considered and is tantamount to achievement. The decisions to split the atom and to place a man on the moon are eloquent sagas illustrating this point. And, the speed with which a commitment will be realized depends upon the priority assigned. As a health care issue, it is a serious mistake to assign less than the highest priority to improving health care of the population as a whole through minority recruitment.

## *AN EXAMPLE OF COMMITMENT FOR CHANGE*

In the early 1970s, the University of California, San Francisco School of Pharmacy, recognizing its responsibilities to *all* the citizens of California, devised a successful strategy of minority recruitment and retention to address one formidable barrier of access to quality pharmaceutical care . . . the absence of minority pharmacy professionals. The strategy developed required the commitment of administration, faculty, and students. The rewards were, over a ten year period, that seventeen minority graduates joined the faculties of Schools of Pharmacy across the nation. Subsequently, importantly, and undeniably that commitment by the UCSF School of Pharmacy increased diversity within our pharmacy faculties.

## *MAKING THE CASE FOR FINANCIAL ASSISTANCE*

Commitment includes providing resources for both recruitment and retention. The need for higher education is just as great among racial and ethnic minorities and the poor as it is in the rest of the population. However, colleges and universities were slow to serve even the most able students in this segment of society. Considerable improvement has occurred over the past twenty years despite the fact that efforts were blunted, and continue to be blunted, by inadequate financial aid. The first and most obvious step in any successful recruitment program is the securing of sufficient funds for financial aid. If recruitment programs are to reach into the low income areas, we will then be reaching students whose families are unable to make significant contributions toward their education. Therefore, it is unrealistic to suggest that those students can pay tuition and other fees. In response, some say that there is a long list of government programs and private philanthropic organizations which provide substantial financial support to economically disadvantaged students. The reality is that the financial pressures the state governments are presently suffering is causing a reordering of priorities and, accordingly, diluting past commitments. As of this writing, the financial picture is becoming increasingly bleak. Therefore, it is incumbent upon our professional associations, whether they be local, state or national, to assist our schools in locating and establishing financial assistance for the underprivileged and the underrepresented. That is commitment.

As an example of commitment for local, state, and regional organizations, one approach would be to make *low interest* loans available by negotiating guarantees either through the associations or in concert with the local bank. The guaranteed federal loans now available are high interest loans, sufficiently high to discourage potential applicants to our schools to pursue an education in pharmacy. One must recognize that most minority students are in the lower incomes strata, usually have little collateral and, therefore, are poor risks for the banking community. Accordingly, evidence of commitment could come in the form of assisting the schools in securing loan funds for high-risk students. Concomitantly, getting involved in an effort to support the negotiation of loan guarantees would aid in the recruitment of the underprivileged and the underrepresented. That, again, would be commitment; an engagement to assume a financial obligation as an expression of support for diversity which, subsequently, would lead to the improvement of the delivery of pharmaceutical care for all the citizens of this country.

Although commitment is the theme of this effort, "Health is our Concern" is, appropriately, the real issue underlying commitment. My concern is whether we will all move forward because more of us will be involved in commitment, or whether our hesitancy in embracing commitment will contribute to the ever-widening gap between the healthy and the ill. We can narrow, even close that gap with the tools we have; education, involvement and commitment.

I trust health care practitioners and educators concur that the opportunity and the responsibility to improve the delivery of health care rests with each of us and also recognize that *commitment* to providing access to an education in pharmacy is part of the equation in solving the problem of the double standard of health care.

## REFERENCES

1. Statement of the Honorable William R. Roy, U.S. House of Representatives. Hearing before the Committee on Ways and Means, House of Representatives, 92nd Congress on national health insurance proposals. 19 Nov. 1971.

2. U.S. Department of Health, Education, and Welfare. Public Health Service. Vital and health statistics data on national health resources. Pharmacy manpower, U.S., 2, 1966.

3. Lee RI, Jones LW. The fundamentals of good medical care. Chicago, IL: University of Chicago Press, 1933.

# Clinical Rotations at a Historically Black College: A Vital Component

Adrian Goram

**SUMMARY.** Pharmacy students graduating from one of the four Historically Black Colleges and Universities (HBCUs) that offers a degree in pharmacy receive an invaluable education not only in pharmacy, but a heightened cultural awareness necessary for a profession within an ethnocentric society. The clinical rotation plays a pivotal role in the pharmacy curriculum. Unlike any other rotation, it actively integrates the didactic skills in an applied clinical setting, as evaluated by the preceptor who also serves as teacher. The role model concept is extremely vital at an HBCU as well as the clinical setting because it is appreciated by all students.

Other important concerns addressed include the issues of recruitment and retention of minority faculty, the misconceptions of HBCUs and the strengths of the clinical rotation as they relate to the needs of the students from the perspective of a new minority faculty member.

As a novice pharmacy faculty member at a Historically Black College or University (HBCU), one of the most rewarding experiences for me is the baccalaureate and commencement ceremonies for our graduating pharmacy students. As a recent graduate from an HBCU, I share their enthusiasm and sense of accomplished goals. More importantly, I see the evolution of many from frustrated, motivatively starved students to confident neophytes with competent pharmacy skills who are eagerly awaiting to start their pharmaceutical career. I feel good about this transition primarily because of my contributions to their education as teacher, counselor, advisor and lastly, preceptor of a clinical rotation.

---

Adrian Goram, Pharm.D., is Assistant Professor of Clinical Pharmacy at the Xavier University of Louisiana College of Pharmacy, New Orleans, LA 70125.

 

The clinical rotation experience represents an important component of the last phase of pharmacy education. All of the 74 accredited colleges/universities offer various lengths of exposure of the clinical pharmacy rotation in their curriculum. Of this number, four pharmacy schools are located on predominantly HBCUs: Howard University, Florida A&M University, Texas Southern University and Xavier University of Louisiana.

In addition to the high quality of education at an HBCU, a firm foundation is provided for ALL students in a nurturing environment enriched with Black heritage and tradition and mentored by a culturally diverse faculty that prepare students for a potentially rewarding profession within an ethnocentric society (1). These principles are well aligned with the philosophies of pharmacy education. This is presumably beneficial because a sense of awareness is instilled about racism and discrimination with which many students will inevitably be confronted. The clinical rotation is designed for the students to integrate actively and improve their knowledge base acquired from the didactic portion of the curriculum while exposed in a clinically academic setting. This article is a commentary on the educational mission of HBCUs, the misconceptions and strengths of the clinical rotation as well as the future expectations of pharmacy education at an HBCU from a new clinical faculty member.

## *THE ROLE OF HBCUs*

There are 117 HBCUs in this country. Of this number, 41 private schools exist under the United Negro College Fund, UNCF (1). As previously stated, four of the 74 accredited pharmacy schools are located at HBCUs. However, Xavier University of Louisiana is the nation's only Catholic HBCU affiliated with UNCF (2).

It is not just the religious background that makes Xavier unique, but the traditional commitment by the administration and faculty to harbor a smaller and more supportive environment that is conducive to the whole educational process for the student (1,2). An example of Xavier's successful strategy of education has been demonstrated with their high percentage of students graduating with math and science degrees, including many who later matriculated to medical and dental schools. This success has been recently documented in the national media (3,4). The College of Pharmacy at Xavier began in 1928 and continues the University's proud educational heritage by graduating 25 percent of all Black pharmacists nationwide (5).

Unlike the traditionally white institutions (TWIs) that heavily recruit scholarly or athletic black students for "window dressing" or token purposes, HBCUs have a genuine interest in graduating black students who are considered by many to be educationally compromised or disadvantaged (1). Frequent episodes of racism at white campuses is a factor that has contributed to the recent rise in enrollment at HBCUs (1). It is not the intention of these institutions to temporarily shelter any student from racism, but merely to function as a support mechanism both socially and academically against the backdrop of the devastating impact of racism (1,6). Another factor in the increased enrollment may be the reduction in federal budget dollars that subsidized college tuition cost (2). At most HBCUs, the necessary strides are made to educate students who may be considered as high risk without jeopardizing the standards (1). This is achieved through intensive teacher-student contact, demonstrated in a much smaller ratio, when compared to that of larger institutions (1,2).

There is an apparent rise in white student enrollment at HBCUs. Contrary to popular belief about this influx occurring overnight, it developed gradually within the past 20 years (6). While many fear the shift in the racial mix will dilute or virtually eliminate the heritage of HBCUs, others aggressively recruit white students at HBCUs (6,7). These educators view this racial mix as an opportunity to destroy misconceptions that regard HBCUs as inferior institutions. Furthermore, it fosters improved communications and respect among all races without compromising the identity and mission of HBCUs (7).

## *THE STRENGTHS OF THE CLINICAL ROTATION*

Mixed feelings are expressed by students once they matriculate to rotations. On the brighter side, students are eligible to graduate once they have completed their hourly requirements on rotations which include exposures to hospital, retail and clinical practice settings. Some students may perceive a rotation as a peaceful transition from the grueling class work. As a result, some students may expect preceptors to be lenient. There are other students who view their time spent on other rotations as inexpensive labor, with very little professional activities encountered. For the conscientious student, a rotation of this kind is nonproductive and more emphasis is placed on the time remaining, rather than the activities performed.

On the clinical rotation, students expect to be challenged, mainly because their preceptors also have been their teachers in clinical didactic courses. Although the clinical faculty may have an idea of the student's performance in the classroom, it may not be directly related to their knowledge skills and hence, their performance on rotations. One of the advantages of the clinical rotation is the small, tutor-intensive . . . approach that develops a higher order thinking necessary in pharmacy practice. This philosophy is paralleled with the mission of HBCUs. One of the methods employed by our clinical faculty is the enhancement of the student's metacognitive processes, as described by Presseison (8). This involves the self-motivation of students to become aware of their learning deficiencies or improve their aptitude as they achieve more autonomy (8).

Another advantage of the clinical rotation is that of observing role models in action. Students appreciate their pharmacy education through the mentorship of the preceptor. Daily clinical activities such as professional duties to medical personnel, require an assertiveness on the pharmacist's part. From past discussions with my clinical colleagues, emphasis has always been placed on the quality of education by the faculty. Students may not be completely color blind, but it is the impression of my colleagues that all students judge minority faculty members by their character and credibility instead of their skin color. It is also my belief that my colleagues show no racial preference to any pharmacy students.

Clinical preceptors also illustrate career options for students. My area of expertise is hematology-oncology. Other areas offered at Xavier include cardiovascular, psychiatry, infectious diseases, pediatrics, geriatrics and ambulatory care. These choices represent diversity within the clinical arena. The ultimate outcome the students should observe is improved patient care with clinical pharmacy intervention. As students participate in these day-to-day activities, it leaves a respectable impression.

It is disturbing to me when pharmacy students have doubts about the profession before their careers start. Therefore, the faculty must seize the opportunity to groom students to consider academia as a potential career path. With the continuing shortage of pharmacists in the nation, students should realize they are in a unique position to harness the satisfaction of pharmacy practice by becoming more patient oriented through counseling and consultation (9). Students also see firsthand the various opportunities in clinical pharmacy.

In short, not only do students develop clinical skills, they begin to appreciate their pharmacy education through the preparational guidance of the preceptor. It is indeed rewarding to know that our curriculum is at least comparable or superior to other pharmacy schools. The experience during the clinical rotation could be a factor that makes students aware and appreciate their pharmacy education from an HBCU retrospectively.

## *RECRUITMENT/RETENTION OF CLINICAL PHARMACY FACULTY*

By the year 2000, more than half a million faculty positions will be available on campuses across the country (10). As senior faculty members retire, it is becoming increasingly difficult for college administrators to replace them (11). Pharmacy faculties are by no means immune to this shortage. Current demographics of the 74 accredited colleges and schools of pharmacy show that only 4.2% of the faculty are Black Americans (12). Surely, a statistic of this kind supports the need to aggressively recruit and retain more black faculty in our pharmacy schools, especially among our HBCUs.

In an article appearing in the *American Journal of Pharmaceutical Education*, Engle describes the female as the new faculty member of the future (13). Albeit true, the issues such as factors that may impede promotion and tenure described in her article could also be applied to the concerns of minority faculty, regardless of gender at an HBCU. As the college age population of students (18-24 years) continues to rise above 25 million by the year 2000, so will the proportionate number of blacks and other minority students. Since many faculty positions are dependent upon student enrollment, the demand for minority faculty is clearly evident (11). While emphasis is and continues to be placed on the recruiting of African-American students at HBCUs, they require the presence of eligible minority faculty as role models to see that an academic career is viable (1,10).

Retention is just as important as recruitment. The factors that keep me in academia are student development and professional growth, as well as optimum patient care. Factors such as these fulfill my need for job satisfaction. Despite my satisfactory needs, these objectives may have different levels of priorities to that of the administrative or rank and tenure bodies. This creates a dilemma when one is evaluated for rank and tenure. This is not isolated just at my institution, but a common complaint registered by many of my clinical colleagues nationwide.

Eligibility for promotion encompasses the never ending art of juggling teaching, scholarly and community activities. Besides the enthusiasm, retention must consider the terms of morale, rewards and commitment. So many questions regarding these issues remain unanswered. This exists primarily because the hierarchy of college of pharmacy faculty do not fit the traditional mold in a liberal arts setting. According to Marcellus Grace, Ph.D. and Dean of Xavier's College of Pharmacy, the faculty growth enables us to be different, not special.

As we embark on the implementation of the all Pharm.D. curriculum, the clinical faculty should be at the forefront as role models for not only students, but our associates as well. The clinical rotation plays a pivotal role in this objective. Moreover, faculty support between clinical and nonclinical personnel should be mutually complementary. As I climb the academic career ladder, I look forward to the support from all my colleagues.

## *CONCLUSION*

Historically, HBCU students experience cultural diversity and begin to appreciate and respect the dignity of all mankind. Although, the clinical rotation is short, it is a major impact on pharmacy education. Additionally, the clinical arena has unlimited areas of growth for the student to consider. The skills the students develop on clinical rotation could be applied at various levels of pharmacy practice. As a graduate and a new clinical faculty member at an HBCU, I can personally appreciate the need for the recruitment and retention of minority faculty members. Without them, the impact of the role model concept is limited.

Nonclinical faculty members also need to understand the clinical faculty member's role in patient care. I suggest an annual day of observation by the basic science faculty. This could possibly explain why more time is spent at individual sites and less time spent on campus. Morale and satisfaction are issues directly related to our interest in the student's well-being and patient care. I also feel that my clinical colleagues would not sacrifice their salary potential in academia if they were not deeply concerned for the students and drug therapy affecting patient care. It is my perspective that racial preference is not the issue, but the quality of education is. It matters when the education comes from an HBCU.

In conclusion, my gratitude is sustained when I see former students gainfully employed in their chosen field of pharmacy, thanks to their invaluable education they received at an HBCU.

## REFERENCES

1. Wiley E. Black students increasingly see HBCUs as institutions of choice. Black Issues Higher Educ 1991; 7(24):9-11.

2. Anon. Rediscovering Black college experience. Xavier Gold 1990;(Winter):41-5.

3. Toch T. Teaching science the hard way. US News World Rep 1990;5:601.

4. Anon. Tiny Black college takes high road in sciences. New York Times 28 Mar 1990.

5. The Xavier Force 1990; (6):1.

6. Wiley E, Hughes M. Historically Black colleges becoming increasingly white. Black Issues Higher Educ 1991; 7(25):28-31.

7. Wiley E. African American educator urges HBCUs to aggressively recruit white students. Black Issues Higher Educ 1991; 7(25):29-31.

8. Jang R, Solad SW. Teaching pharmacy students problem-solving: theory and present status. Am J Pharm Educ 1990; 54:161-6.

9. Brody R. Does it pay to be a pharmacist? Am Druggist 1991; (Feb):36- 45.

10. Mercer J. Support, encouragement required to increase number of Black faculty. Black Issues Higher Educ 1990; 7(22):30-2.

11. Hocker C. In search of Black faculty. Black Enterprise 1991; 10(20):70-6.

12. Meyer SM, Sherman MS. 1990-1991 profile of pharmacy faculty. Alexandria, VA: American Association of Colleges of Pharmacy.

13. Engle JP. Profile of the new faculty member of the future. Am J Pharm Educ 1990; 54:363-5.

# Cooperative Approaches to Stimulating Minority Participation in Graduate Pharmaceutical Education

Michael C. Gerald
John M. Cassady

**SUMMARY.** There exists a paucity of minority students in higher education in general and in graduate pharmaceutical education in particular. A formal articulation has been created between the Colleges of Pharmacy of The Ohio State University and Xavier University of Louisiana, majority and minority institutions, respectively. This agreement has as its primary objective to stimulate undergraduate minority student interest and promote their participation in graduate and postbaccalaureate professional pharmaceutical education. It also provides for the exchange of visiting professors between the institutions. The provisions of this agreement and the progress to date are described.

Blacks, Hispanics, and American Indians are underrepresented in post-graduate higher education, a pattern observed in professional education and graduate programs in science, engineering, and pharmacy. This paucity of graduate students is directly responsible for the insufficient numbers of minority pharmacy faculty members and scientists. To contribute to the alleviation of this problem, a linkage was established between Xavier–an institution providing a source of qualified undergraduate mi-

---

Michael C. Gerald, Ph.D., is Associate Dean and Professor of Pharmacology and John M. Cassady, Ph.D., is Dean and Professor of Medicinal Chemistry and Pharmacognosy at the Ohio State University College of Pharmacy, 500 West 12th Avenue, Columbus, OH 43210.

Permission to use the Affiliation Agreement between Ohio State University and Xavier University of Louisiana (appendix) is granted from Xavier University of Louisiana College of Pharmacy.

 

nority students and Ohio State–an institution seeking to play a proactive role in providing graduate pharmaceutical education to underrepresented minorities. To further this objective, a formal articulation agreement has been developed between these institutions, the provisions of which are described here and which may serve as a model for other similar joint ventures between majority and minority institutions. This paper describes such a cooperative and symbiotic relationship and concludes with an appraisal of our progress to date.

The paper begins by presenting a global overview of the participation of minorities in higher education to offer a context for better understanding the demographics of minorities in pharmacy education.

## *DEMOGRAPHICS OF MINORITIES IN HIGHER EDUCATION*

A superficial perusal of the demographic statistics of minority participation in higher education suggests that considerable advances were made between the late 1970s and 1980s. Increases of 30.9 and 63.4 percent in the numbers of bachelor's and first-professional degrees awarded, respectively, were noted from 1976 to 1987. At the doctorate level, minorities earned 7.6 percent more Ph.D.s in 1988 than in 1978 (Table 1) (1).

More critical analysis of these numbers reveals significant imbalances among racial/ethnic groups and between genders. These differences become evident when we examine the parity relationship between the proportion of a racial/ethnic group participating in a degree category and the fraction of the national population represented by that group. When so expressed, whites are proportionately represented, with those receiving bachelor's, master's, doctorate, and first-professional degrees constituting 94-106 percent of their numbers in the population. With the exception of Asian-Americans who earn degrees at a proportion which constitutes up to 127 percent of their representation in the population, other minority groups are underrepresented across degree categories: blacks, 28.5-46.3 percent; Hispanics, 29.6-35.8 percent; and American-Indians, 57.1 percent (Table 1).

Of all racial/ethnic groups, blacks–in particular, black males–experienced the greatest decreases in all degree categories from the period of 1976-78 to 1987-88. The overall 4.3 percent reduction in blacks earning bachelor's degrees, and in particular, the 12.2 percent decrease among black males, portends a significant attenuation in the pipeline of individuals subsequently eligible to enter graduate programs. Blacks also experi-

## TABLE 1. Population and Earned Degrees by Race/Ethnicity and Sex[1]

| | United States Population[2] | | Bachelor's | | Master's | | Doctorates[3] | | First Professional | |
|---|---|---|---|---|---|---|---|---|---|---|
| | %1988 Total | 1988 vs 1980[4] | %1987 Total | 1987 vs 1976 | %1987 Total | 1987 vs 1976 | %1987 Total | 1988 vs 1978 | %1987 Total | 1987 vs 1976 |
| **Total** | 100.0 | 8.2 | 100.0 | 7.9 | 100.0 | -6.4 | 100.0 | -8.4 | 100.0 | 15.4 |
| men | | | 48.5 | -3.8 | 48.8 | -14.6 | 59.0 | -23.8 | 65.0 | -11.2 |
| women | | | 51.5 | 21.9 | 51.2 | -3.0 | 41.0 | 29.2 | 35.0 | 158.2 |
| **Minority** | 15.8 | 19.9 | 12.1 | 30.9 | 10.6 | 0.5 | 9.1 | 7.6 | 11.2 | 63.4 |
| men | | | 11.3 | 23.6 | 10.1 | 4.7 | 8.0 | -11.5 | 10.2 | 23.2 |
| women | | | 12.9 | 37.6 | 11.0 | -2.9 | 10.7 | 40.4 | 13.2 | 206.7 |
| **Asian** | 2.6 | 70.3 | 3.3 | 191.4 | 3.0 | 118.8 | 2.6 | 56.9 | 3.2 | 135.9 |
| men | | | 3.6 | 173.0 | 3.7 | 117.4 | 3.0 | 43.9 | 3.1 | 88.6 |
| women | | | 3.0 | 215.3 | 2.2 | 121.1 | 2.1 | 93.2 | 3.4 | 306.2 |
| **Black** | 12.3 | 12.7 | 5.7 | -4.3 | 4.8 | -31.8 | 3.5 | -22.1 | 4.8 | 26.9 |
| men | | | 4.7 | -12.2 | 3.6 | -34.0 | 2.3 | 46.7 | 3.9 | -8.9 |
| women | | | 6.7 | 1.7 | 5.9 | -30.5 | 5.2 | 10.0 | 6.3 | 133.8 |
| **Hispanic[5]** | 8.1 | 34.1 | 2.7 | 50.3 | 2.4 | 32.9 | 2.6 | 25.6 | 2.9 | 90.1 |
| men | | | 2.7 | 26.5 | 2.4 | 16.1 | 2.3 | 1.3 | 2.8 | 42.4 |
| women | | | 2.8 | 81.3 | 2.5 | 52.8 | 2.9 | 75.0 | 3.0 | 356.1 |
| **Amer-Indian** | 0.7 | 18.9 | 0.4 | 13.6 | 0.4 | 41.4 | 0.4 | 55.0 | 0.4 | 60.8 |
| men | | | 0.4 | -5.0 | 0.4 | 21.3 | 0.4 | 2.0 | 0.4 | 12.9 |
| women | | | 0.4 | 36.1 | 0.4 | 65.9 | 0.4 | 320.0 | 0.5 | 365.4 |
| **White** | 84.2 | 6.2 | 84.9 | 3.7 | 79.1 | -12.9 | 89.3 | -5.2 | 87.5 | 11.3 |
| men | | | 84.6 | -8.5 | 74.7 | 24.3 | 90.0 | -21.0 | 88.4 | -13.9 |
| women | | | 85.2 | 18.6 | 83.3 | 0 | 88.3 | 34.5 | 85.8 | 153.0 |

1 Earned degree data from reference (1)
2 U.S. Department of Commerce, Bureau of Census, series P.25, No.1045.
3 U.S. citizens only.
4 Expressed as a percent change for the years noted.
5 Persons of Hispanic origin may be of any race; the majority are included as white.

enced a 22.1 percent decrease in the numbers of doctorates earned from 1978 to 1988, with black males declining by 46.7 percent.

Proportionately fewer blacks enrolled as undergraduates are earning bachelor's degrees than are whites. A comparison of students enrolled in 1986 with degrees earned in 1987 reveals that while blacks represented 9.2 percent of the undergraduate population in 1986, only 5.7 percent graduated the following year. By contrast, 79.2 percent of all 1986 undergraduates were white and yet whites constituted 87.5 percent of all bachelor's graduates in 1987 (1).

Hispanics (1), in contrast to blacks, made significant gains in the number of degrees earned between 1976 and 1987: bachelor's, 50.3 percent increase; master's, 32.9 percent; doctorate, 25.6 percent; and first-professional degree, 90.1 percent. By a significant margin, greater gains were made by Hispanic women than men (Table 1).

By far, Asian-Americans are proportionately best represented in higher education and have exhibited the greatest gains among minority racial/ethnic categories in degrees earned from 1976 to 1987: bachelor's, 215.3 percent increase; master's, 121.1 percent; doctorate, 93.2 percent; and first-professional degree, 306.2 percent. Although as in other categories females showed greater growth than males, the disparity was somewhat less disproportionate with Asian Americans.

At all levels of higher education, American Indians only earn about 0.4 percent of degrees granted. Gains in the percentage of degrees earned from 1976 to 1987 were seen across all degree levels, with women primarily responsible for the gains in almost all instances.

Major differences are observed among racial/ethnic groups in their selection of fields for advanced training. This impact is particularly felt in the sciences and engineering (2). Significant numbers of underrepresented minority students (i.e., blacks, Hispanics, American Indians) drop out of science early in high school. This results in a poor foundation in mathematics and science and contributes to the fewer number of such students entering science-oriented majors in college. Other contributing factors include a lack of orientation to pursue higher education and the severe shortage of role models and mentors.

Underrepresented minorities currently constitute 22 percent of our population but only 4.4 percent of scientists and engineers. Among 1,268 Ph.D. degrees awarded to U.S. citizens in 1989, only 65 (5 percent) were earned by Hispanics and blacks. The number of Ph.D. degrees granted to blacks has not increased since 1975; the highest percentage increases have occurred among Asian-Americans and Hispanics (2).

A composite summary of the racial/ethnic demographics of instructional faculty in all institutions of higher education is presented in Table 2 (3). These data may be compared with the proportion of the various racial/ethnic groups within the total population. Minority members of the population are generally underrepresented as instructional faculty. Of all instructional faculty, 10.1 percent are members of a racial/ethnic minority, only 63.9 percent of their representation in the population. Black faculty members are represented at one-third parity, whereas Hispanics and American-Indian faculty members represent 21.0 percent and 57.1 percent, respectively, of their ethnic group's contribution to the population. Asian-American faculty are represented at 154 percent of their numbers in the general population, whereas whites are closest to parity at 107 percent.

Comparisons may also be made between numbers of those from minority groups enrolled as students and serving as faculty. The overall percentage of minority faculty members (10.1 percent) is comparable to the proportion of minority students (9.1-11.2 percent) enrolled in master's, doctorate, and first-professional degree programs but lower than the percentage (12.1 percent) enrolled for the bachelor's degree. Blacks and Asian Americans each constitute about four percent of the total instructional faculty. It is beyond the scope of this paper to attempt to further analyze the racial/ethnic distribution among academic disciplines or across levels of higher education.

This situation has prompted many national professional and education-

TABLE 2. Comparative Racial/Ethnic Demographics of Instructional Faculty

| | All Institutions[1] | | | Colleges of Pharmacy[2] | | |
|---|---|---|---|---|---|---|
| | N | % | | N | % | |
| Total | 464,072 | 100.0 | | 2939 | 100.0 | |
| Minority | 47,036 | 10.1 | [63.9][3] | 385 | 13.1 | [82.9] |
| Asian | 18,370 | 4.0 | [154] | 186 | 6.3 | [242] |
| Black | 19,227 | 4.1 | [33.3] | 122 | 4.2 | [34.1] |
| Hispanic[4] | 7,704 | 1.7 | [33.3] | 64 | 2.2 | [27.2] |
| Amer-Indian | 1,735 | 0.4 | [57.1] | 13 | 0.4 | [57.1] |
| White | 417,036 | 89.9 | [107] | 2554 | 86.9 | [103] |

[1]Full-time instructional faculty in all institutions of higher education in 1985 (Reference 3).

[2]Paid full-time and part-time faculty in 74 colleges of pharmacy in 1990-91 for which race/ethnicity has been reported (Reference 7).

[3]Expression of parity (where 100 = parity): percent of racial-ethnicity category as instructional faculty/percent of category in total population (Table 1).

[4]Persons of Hispanic origin may be of any race.

al organizations and universities to develop programs to increase minority participation in graduate programs. Some of these programs, including the new National Science Foundation initiative, are comprehensive from K-12 to college and through graduate studies. This program, with recruitment activities focused on minority students, has established a turn of the century goal of increasing to 2,000 the number of Ph.D.s granted to minority U.S. citizens (2). Other programs include locator services, summer research opportunities, faculty and student exchanges between minority and majority institutions, and graduate recruitment conferences and fairs. Involvement of minority students in the recruitment process is thought to be useful (4).

## *DEMOGRAPHICS OF MINORITIES IN PHARMACY EDUCATION*

Undergraduate studies in pharmacy provide an excellent preparation for many pharmacy graduate programs and, in some cases (for example, the postbaccalaureate doctor of pharmacy degree), the only acceptable prerequisite background. From 1972 to 1989, the overall percentage of entry-level professional pharmacy degrees (B.S. and Pharm.D.) awarded to minority students increased from 8.7 to 15.1 percent (Table 3) (5).

More critical analysis of the data reveals that these gains were primarily attributed to a 2.3-fold increase in the numbers of Asian-Americans and a 1.9-fold increase in blacks–in particular, black females–earning degrees during these years. This gender differential was most apparent after 1980. Between 1981 and 1989, there were 77.6 and 22.9 percent more B.S. and entry-level Pharm.D. black female graduates, respectively, than males (5). The average numbers of entry-level Hispanic students graduating from the period 1972-75 to 1986-89 increased by 29.4 percent. Although American Indians are only modestly represented in pharmacy programs, student enrollment has risen significantly from 45 to 81 from 1987 to 1989 (6). Despite these gains, we should not lose sight of the fact that considerable disparity continues to exist between their participation in these programs and their representation in the population.

Academic posts and leadership positions in industry and government generally require that candidates have an earned terminal degree (i.e., Ph.D., Pharm.D.) and, to an increasing extent, postdoctoral training. Disappointingly few blacks, Hispanics, and American-Indians earn Ph.D. degrees in the pharmaceutical sciences, with their sum total rarely in

TABLE 3. Entry-Level Pharmacy Degrees (B.S., Pharm. D.) Conferred by Minority Racial/Ethnic Group, 1972-1989[1]

| | Asian American | Black | Hispanic | American Indian | Total Minority/period | Total Degrees/period[2] |
|---|---|---|---|---|---|---|
| 1972–1975 | | | | | | |
| Total/period | 613[4] | 600 | 751 | 15 | 1979 | 22,711 |
| Average/year | 204.3 | 150.0 | 187.8 | 5.0 | 547.1 | 5677.8 |
| Range/year | 188–219 | 138–176 | 134–272 | 0–8 | | 4858–6712 |
| % Total[3] | 2.7 | 2.6 | 3.3 | 0.07 | 8.7 | |
| 1976–1980 | | | | | | |
| Total/period | 1264 | 1162 | 1414 | 49 | 3889 | 38,248 |
| Average/year | 252.8 | 232.4 | 282.8 | 9.8 | 777.8 | 7649.6 |
| Range/year | 222–292 | 226–272 | 241–315 | 6–15 | | 7432–8011 |
| % Total | 3.3 | 3.0 | 3.7 | 0.13 | 10.2 | |
| 1981–1985 | | | | | | |
| Total/period | 1580 | 1213 | 1225 | 42 | 4060 | 32,254 |
| Average/year | 316.0 | 242.6 | 245.0 | 8.4 | 812.0 | 6450.8 |
| Range/year | 288–339 | 230–250 | 217–261 | 5–13 | | 5735–7323 |
| % Total | 4.9 | 3.8 | 3.8 | 0.13 | 12.6 | |
| 1986–1989 | | | | | | |
| Total/period | 1480 | 1196 | 972 | 43 | 3691 | 24,395 |
| Average/year | 370.0 | 299 | 243.0 | 10.8 | 922.8 | 6098.8 |
| Range/year | 335–454 | 282–310 | 217–258 | 8–12 | | 5800–6557 |
| % Total | 6.1 | 4.9 | 4.0 | 0.18 | 15.1 | |

1 Reference (5).
2 Degrees conferred to all graduates.
3 Percentage of total degrees conferred to minorities/period.
4 1973-1975 only.

excess of four percent of doctoral degrees earned by all American students (Table 4). Since 1972 on only two occasions have as many as four black students and on only four instances have at least four Hispanic students earned this terminal science degree in a given year; since 1987 Hispanics have been exhibiting a generally improving trend (5). By contrast, Asian-Americans consistently receive more than half the total of all Ph.D. degrees earned by minority students in pharmacy.

An entry-level professional pharmacy degree is often used as undergraduate preparation for doctoral studies in the pharmaceutical sciences. When the numbers of Ph.D. degrees earned from 1986-1989 are expressed as percentages of entry-level professional degrees earned by specific racial/ethnic groups, we see a rank order of Asian-Americans and whites (each 2.4 percent), Hispanics (1.2 percent), and blacks (0.84 percent) (5). With regard to the percentage of postbaccalaureate Pharm.D. degrees awarded to American students, among minority categories during the 1980s blacks fared best, followed by Asian-Americans and Hispanics (Table 5).

Members of minority groups appear to be proportionately better represented on college of pharmacy faculties than institutions of higher education taken as a whole, i.e., 82.9 versus 63.9 percent of group population parity (7). This difference may be principally accounted for by the greater representation of Asian-American (242 percent of group population parity) and a small contribution by Hispanic (27.2 percent) faculty members in pharmacy schools (Table 2). While it may be argued that the 1990-91 data for pharmacy faculty cannot be compared directly with 1985 data for all faculty, it is unclear that substantive quantitative demographic changes have occurred in the intervening years that would significantly alter the conclusions presented.

## *OBJECTIVES OF THE OHIO STATE-XAVIER COOPERATIVE VENTURE*

The objectives of the Ohio State-Xavier venture were driven by an overall philosophical societal commitment by The Ohio State University. As a public land grant institution, Ohio State is deeply committed to a societal responsibility to provide access to students of all racial and ethnic origins. The University has an aggressive affirmative action program that seeks to enroll (and, more importantly, graduate) underrepresented minority students at all levels including postbaccalaureate graduate and professional studies in the health sciences.

TABLE 4. Ph.D. Degrees in the Pharmaceutical Sciences Conferred by Minority Racial/Ethnic Group, 1972-1989[1]

| | Asian American | Black | Hispanic | American Indian | Total Minority | Total American | Total Degrees[2] |
|---|---|---|---|---|---|---|---|
| 1972-1975 | | | | | | | |
| Total/period | 15 | 11 | 6 | 0 | 32 | 511 | 728 |
| Average/year | 3.8 | 2.8 | 1.5 | 0 | 8.0 | 127.8 | 182.0 |
| Range/year | 3-7 | 2-4 | 1-4 | 0 | | 120-137 | 168-189 |
| % Total[3] | 2.9 | 2.2 | 1.2 | 0 | 6.3 | 100 | |
| 1976-1980 | | | | | | | |
| Total/period | 43 | 7 | 4 | 1 | 55 | 620 | 875 |
| Average/year | 8.6 | 1.4 | 0.8 | 0.2 | 11.0 | 124.0 | 175.0 |
| Range/year | 5-12 | 1-3 | 1 | 0-1 | | 107-144 | 153-189 |
| % Total | 4.9 | 0.8 | 0.5 | 0.11 | 6.3 | 100 | |
| 1981-1985 | | | | | | | |
| Total/period | 73 | 6 | 12 | 1 | 62 | 739 | 1029 |
| Average/year | 8.6 | 1.2 | 2.4 | 0.2 | 12.4 | 147.8 | 205.8 |
| Range/year | 3-13 | 1-2 | 1-7 | 0-1 | | 132-163 | 180-232 |
| % Total | 5.8 | 0.8 | 1.6 | 0.14 | 8.4 | 100 | |
| 1986-1989 | | | | | | | |
| Total/period | 35 | 10 | 12 | 0 | 57 | 694 | 1093 |
| Average/year | 8.8 | 2.5 | 3.0 | 0 | 14.3 | 173.5 | 273.3 |
| Range/year | 6-13 | 2-4 | 1-4 | 0 | | 158-189 | 260-287 |
| % Total | 5.0 | 1.4 | 1.7 | 0 | 8.2 | 100 | |

1 Reference (5).
2 Degrees conferred to all graduates.
3 Percentage of degrees conferred to all American graduates.

TABLE 5. Postbaccalaureate Pharm. D. Degrees Conferred by Minority Racial/Ethnic Group, 1973-1989[1]

| | Asian American | Black | Hispanic | American Indian | Total Minority | Total American | Total Degrees[2] |
|---|---|---|---|---|---|---|---|
| 1973-1975 | | | | | | | |
| Total/period | 18 | 11 | 1 | 0 | 30 | 370 | 393 |
| Average/year | 6.0 | 3.7 | 0.33 | 0 | 7.5 | 123.3 | 131.0 |
| Range/year | 5-7 | 2.5 | 0-1 | 0 | | 114-132 | 117-140 |
| % Total[3] | 4.9 | 3.0 | 0.27 | 0 | 8.1 | 100 | |
| 1976-1980 | | | | | | | |
| Total/period | 20 | 15 | 7 | 0 | 42 | 840 | 872 |
| Average/year | 4.0 | 3.0 | 1.4 | 0 | 8.4 | 168.0 | 174.4 |
| Range/year | 1-7 | 0-4 | 0-2 | 0 | | 121-185 | 126-190 |
| % Total | 2.4 | 1.8 | 0.83 | 0 | 5.0 | 100 | |
| 1981-1985 | | | | | | | |
| Total/period | 38 | 59 | 26 | 2 | 125 | 1138 | 1243 |
| Average/year | 7.6 | 11.8 | 5.2 | 0.4 | 25.0 | 227.6 | 248.6 |
| Range/year | 3-8 | 6-23 | 2-9 | 0-1 | | 191-295 | 159-222 |
| % Total | 3.3 | 5.2 | 2.3 | 0.18 | 11.0 | 100 | |
| 1986-1989 | | | | | | | |
| Total/period | 29 | 34 | 24 | 0 | 87 | 703 | 803 |
| Average/year | 7.3 | 8.5 | 6.0 | 0 | 21.8 | 175.8 | 200.8 |
| Range/year | 3-14 | 5-15 | 2-9 | 0 | | 133-197 | 159-222 |
| % Total | 4.1 | 4.8 | 3.4 | 0 | 12.4 | 100 | |

[1]Reference (5).
[2]Degrees conferred to all graduates.
[3]Percentage of degrees conferred to all American graduates.

Between the years 1983-1987, Ohio State ranked third nationally in the total numbers of doctor of philosophy degrees earned by blacks and Asian-Americans (8). From 1982-1990, the University conferred a total of 1,146 master's and 308 doctorate degrees to racial/ethnic minorities: black, 687 and 164, respectively; Asian-American/Pacific Islander, 260 and 97; Hispanic, 169 and 41; and American Indian/Alaskan Native, 30 and 6 (9).

Three target objectives were established for the Ohio State-Xavier venture, each of which is independent and not reliant on the success or degree of progress made in meeting the other objectives; these were targets having an impact on students, faculty, and the institution. The participants in this project did not seek nor anticipate achieving a "quick-fix" to alleviating the underrepresented participation of, in this case, blacks in postbaccalaureate pharmaceutical education. Rather the administrations of both institutions sought to develop mutual confidence between the faculties and long-term programmatic support and agreed to share expenses associated with the program.

### *Student Recruitment*

The primary objective is to stimulate and promote minority student interest in postbaccalaureate graduate (M.S., Ph.D.) and professional (Pharm.D.) pharmaceutical education. Although not expressly stated in the articulation agreement, selected minority students who had gained their doctoral degrees at Ohio State, and completed postdoctoral training at another institution, might be recruited to join our faculty.

### *Faculty Interactions*

To develop and encourage collaborative research and scholarly projects of mutual interest between interested faculty at both institutions. This objective was best promoted by providing administrative support for the exchange of visiting professors.

### *Institutional Objectives*

Among the publicly articulated long-range goals of the College of Pharmacy at Ohio State is to increase the numbers of underrepresented minority individuals (in particular, blacks, Hispanics) with doctoral degrees in the health professions and in the pharmaceutical sciences who can contribute to and assume leadership positions in academia, industry, and government. Xavier is committed to assisting Ohio State in its recruiting efforts to achieve this objective.

## *ARTICULATION AGREEMENT BETWEEN THE COLLEGES OF PHARMACY, OF THE OHIO STATE UNIVERSITY AND XAVIER UNIVERSITY OF LOUISIANA*

### *Mechanical Aspects of Establishing Agreement*

Informal discussions by deans at the two institutions revealed a fundamental and mutual desire and commitment to work cooperatively to increase the numbers of underrepresented minority students in postbaccalaureate pharmaceutical education. Although it was acknowledged that a formal agreement between the institutions was highly desirable, there was clear recognition that the success of this relationship was dependent upon the continued goodwill and commitment of the college administration and faculty.

Multiple early drafts of the agreement were exchanged between the parties at the college level to ensure that the basic elements of the informal discussions were captured in the document. Nonbinding and helpful input was solicited from the Provost's office at Ohio State prior to the formal drafting of an articulation agreement. Primary concern focused upon the associated potential binding commitments and obligations. These fears were assuaged by the inclusion of the agreement's preambular statement that "The individual sections of this articulation agreement are based on the availability of suitable faculty members or students and the mutual agreement of both parties to accept such exchange individuals." The document became finalized in Spring 1989 after signatures were secured from the college deans and the vice presidents for academic affairs at both institutions.

### *Overview of the Terms of the Agreement*

The agreement (reproduced in its entirety in the appendix) contains four primary sections: visiting faculty; graduate student recruitment; undergraduate research participation; and the establishment of coordination committees.

*Visiting Faculty*. The agreement describes the duration of faculty visits; fiscal obligations for both institutions, the faculty participants, and sponsors; faculty responsibilities associated with the visit; and the nature of the faculty selection process. Visiting Xavier professors at Ohio State are expected to participate in a research/scholarly project on a full-time basis during 2-4 month appointment periods and provide a final report summarizing the results obtained. Ideally, such relationships would be maintained after the conclusion of the period of the visiting professorship. This individual may also assist the host institution in their undergraduate and graduate minority student initiatives. Such activities might include making recruitment presentations to and meeting with current and prospective students. Financial expenses associated with the leave are to be shared by both institutions.

Visiting Ohio State professors at Xavier are expected to provide scientific or professional seminars to the student body and faculty; consult or collaborate on academic or research projects; and stimulate interest in graduate studies in the pharmaceutical sciences and the postbaccalaureate doctor of pharmacy program.

*Graduate Student Recruitment.* Ohio State faculty will be invited to Xavier to provide general information about its postbaccalaureate professional and graduate studies, including a description of the programs and degree requirements, academic preparation, admission criteria, financial aids, and career opportunities. While obviously highly desirous of attracting Xavier students to Ohio State, we envisioned this objective in a broader context to be the general promotion of postbaccalaureate education. Several primary approaches were adopted to achieve the student recruitment objective as described below.

*Ohio State Recruitment Visits.* One or more Ohio State faculty members visit the Xavier campus for several days each year. Activities associated with this visit include the presentation of a scientific or professional seminar on a topic of interest to the undergraduate pharmacy students; meetings with interested students; and group and individual descriptions of opportunities for postbaccalaureate studies at Ohio State. This visit is scheduled to permit the faculty member to represent the graduate programs at Ohio State at the annual Xavier Graduate and Professional School Day Program.

*Xavier Student Visits to Ohio State.* During the academic year, Xavier students interested in exploring postbaccalaureate educational opportunities at Ohio State are encouraged to visit our College and meet with faculty members and graduate students in their area(s) of interest. They also meet with representatives of the Graduate School and Office of Minority Affairs and tour Columbus.

*Undergraduate Research Participation (URP) Program.* Since 1986,

Ohio State's College of Pharmacy has been recognized as a University Center of Excellence and has received funding from the State of Ohio to promote research and to interest and encourage students to pursue graduate studies in the pharmaceutical sciences. Under the terms of the articulation agreement intended to promote minority student interest in post-baccalaureate pharmacy education, Xavier publicizes Ohio State's annual summer URP program and encourages interested students to make application. Every effort is made to permit student participation on a research/scholarly problem of first choice from among a list of approximately 50 problems. Upon the recommendation of the Xavier pharmacy dean, each year Ohio State will allocate up to two of its 15 positions to Xavier minority pharmacy students. Stipends and housing allowances are provided.

*Coordination Committees.* The agreement calls for the establishment of a joint articulation committee to review the activities described in the articulation agreement and propose changes for future agreements. In addition, the Xavier dean serves as a consultant to Ohio State's College of Pharmacy on affirmative action activities and as an ex officio member of the Ohio State Dean's Advisory Committee on Affirmative Action. Dean Marcellus Grace, Xavier, regularly receives and comments upon the minutes of these Committee meetings and has generously provided our College advice and support in our efforts to recruit minority students.

## APPRAISAL OF PROGRAM PROGRESS

The most important accomplishment of the joint venture to date has been a solidification of goodwill between the faculty and administration of the Colleges of Pharmacy at Ohio State and Xavier. We recognize that both parties are committed to the long-term success of the joint venture and that tangible "bottom line" success will be slow in coming.

### *Faculty Interactions*

During 1990, a Xavier visiting professor spent the summer at Ohio State working on a research problem in medicinal chemistry and utilizing specialized instrumentation available at our college. Both the visiting professor and his host were extremely pleased with their joint venture, the results of which were presented at an international meeting. On the basis of the experience gained on this project, and to support the continuation of this promising research, Xavier purchased a similar nuclear magnetic resonance spectrometer. A member of Xavier's clinical faculty has visited Ohio State, presented a seminar to faculty and students and met with the members of the Student National Pharmaceutical Association, the minority professional organization.

### *Student Recruitment*

Since the program's inception, a total of eight Xavier undergraduates, a member of their staff, and faculty escorts have visited Ohio State in two field trips. The prospective graduate students participated in group orientation programs and for the majority of their time, were hosted by and dined with Ohio State faculty members and students representing academic programs of their greatest interest. Of these, one application was completed and a graduate fellowship was offered. A second individual, while not completing an application, explored two of Ohio State's graduate programs in considerable detail. After much deliberation, these outstanding candidates decided to pursue their graduate studies at other colleges of pharmacy. Some of the undergraduate student visitors were in their early years of professional study, and it is premature to expect their application to our postbaccalaureate programs.

During two successive years, members of the Ohio State faculty have visited the College of Pharmacy at Xavier, presented scholarly seminars, meeting with their faculty and undergraduate students, and attempting to promote linkages between the institutions. The names of pharmacy and nonpharmacy students interested in Ohio State graduate and professional programs were forwarded to the appropriate program personnel.

### *Undergraduate Research Participation Program*

Although a number of students have expressed interest in participating in our summer research program–perhaps as the result of their heightened awareness stimulated by the Ohio State-Xavier interaction–none have participated in our program. Several have pursued similar opportunities at other colleges of pharmacy and in the pharmaceutical industry.

### *Institutional Objectives*

The articulation agreement signed between Ohio State and Xavier has generated considerable interest as a model at Ohio State and in pharmacy education circles (10). The University's higher administration has pointed to it as an exemplar for establishing formal college or departmental agreements between majority and minority institutions. From the outset, both the parties concurred that our relationship would not preclude the entrance into similar agreements with other institutions. Employing the terms of the Xavier agreement, Ohio State is hosting a visiting professor from another minority institution during summer 1991. For its part, Xavier has established similar or identical articulation agreements with the pharmacy schools at the University of Iowa and the University of North Carolina and is in advanced stages of discussion with several other institutions.

Institutions contemplating entering into such relationships should recognize and appreciate that even under the best circumstances and goodwill tangible evidence of progress will be slow in coming and difficult to document. We are hopeful that this long-term investment will result in a significant increase in the numbers of minority graduate students who will provide leadership into the twenty-first century.

## ACKNOWLEDGMENTS

Ohio State College of Pharmacy colleagues Hazel Benson located most useful background material and Kenneth M. Hale generously provided most helpful and constructive comments on this manuscript. The authors recognize the efforts of past-Deans Albert H. Soloway and Dev Pathak in formative stages of discussion with Xavier University about establishing a relationship between Ohio State and Xavier.

## NOTE

1. Persons of Hispanic origin may be of any race. For census purposes, the majority are "white."

## REFERENCES

1. American Council on Education. Minorities in higher education: eighth annual status report, 1989. Washington, DC: American Council on Education, 1989.

2. Rawls RL. Minorities in science. C&EN 1991;69(15):20-35.

3. United States Equal Employment Opportunity Commission. Higher education staff information report file, 1985 (unpublished data).

4. Olson C. Recruiting and retaining minority graduate students: a systems perspective. J Negro Educ 1988;57:31-42.

5. Penna RP, Sherman MS. Degrees conferred by schools and colleges of pharmacy, 1988-1989. Am J Pharm Educ 1990;54:304-19.

6. Penna RP, Sherman MS. Enrollments in schools and colleges of pharmacy, 1988-1989. Am J Pharm Educ 1990;54:451-77.

7. American Association of Colleges of Pharmacy. Profile of pharmacy faculty, 1990-1991. Alexandria, VA: American Association of Colleges of Pharmacy.

8. Office of Scientific and Engineering Personnel. National Research Council. Summary report 1987: doctorate recipients from United States universities. Washington, DC: National Academy Press, 1989.

9. Edgar A. Ohio State University Graduate School, 1991 (unpublished data).

10. Gerald MC, Cassady JM, Grace M. Ohio State-Xavier agreement for graduate and faculty collaborative ventures. American Association of Colleges of Pharmacy abstracts of podium and poster sessions, 1989

# APPENDIX

## Articulation Agreement Between the Colleges of Pharmacy of The Ohio State University and Xavier University of Louisiana

The individual sections of this articulation agreement are based on the availability of suitable faculty members or students and the mutual agreement of both parties to accept such individuals.

## *I. VISITING FACULTY*

### *A. Duration*

This agreement establishes the reciprocal exchange of visiting professors between The Ohio State University and Xavier University of Louisiana no fewer than once during successive 12 month periods.

1. The Ohio State University College of Pharmacy will sponsor the visit of one Xavier University of Louisiana visiting professor annually. It is generally envisioned that such visits will be during the summer and one quarter/semester/term (3-4 months) in duration; based upon mutual consent this period may be shorter or longer and during a time other than the summer. Activities associated with this visit may be pursued prior to or after the actual period of residence in Columbus.

2. A faculty member from The Ohio State University College of Pharmacy will visit the Xavier University of Louisiana campus (e.g., to teach a minicourse, consult or collaborate on academic or research projects, discuss opportunities for graduate and post-baccalaureate study at The Ohio State University College of Pharmacy) for a mutually acceptable period of time. Xavier University of Louisiana will assist in arranging housing.

### *B. Fiscal Considerations*

1. The professor will be granted a professional leave from Xavier University of Louisiana College of Pharmacy which will be responsible for providing salary, fringe benefits, and traveling expenses.

2. The Ohio State University College of Pharmacy will assist in arranging housing and will be responsible for providing a reasonable allowance to defray housing expenses while in Columbus ($1000/month). The Ohio State University College of Pharmacy will provide the equipment and laboratory or office space required to carry out the project. The director of the sponsoring project at The Ohio State University will provide all research supplies.

### *C. Responsibilities*

1. The visiting professor will participate on a research/scholarly project on essentially a full-time basis. The specific nature of the project will be based upon the mutual agreement of the visiting professor and the sponsoring division or professor of The Ohio State University. A final report summarizing the results of the project will be submitted to the deans of the Colleges of Pharmacy of The Ohio State University and Xavier University of Louisiana.

2. The visiting professor will assist The Ohio State University in its undergraduate or graduate minority recruitment efforts by providing consultation with its faculty and administration, and making presentations to and meeting with current and prospective undergraduate and graduate students.

### *D. Selection Process*

1. With the support of the Xavier University of Louisiana Dean, the visiting professor, specializing in the pharmaceutical sciences or pharma-

cy practice, will formally apply to The Ohio State University College of Pharmacy and the sponsoring division.

2. The Ohio State University College of Pharmacy and sponsoring division and faculty member(s), after reviewing the letter of application, resume of the candidate, and the proposed nature of the research/scholarly activity, may agree to serve as sponsors of the visiting professor and the proposed project. In addition, they may agree to provide reasonable space, facilities, equipment, and supplies that are required to successfully pursue the project.

## *II. GRADUATE STUDENT RECRUITMENT*

### *A. The Ohio State University Recruitment Visits*

1. Once annually, for a recommended 3-5 working days, The Ohio State University faculty member will be invited to present a scientific or professional lecture (on a topic acceptable to Xavier University of Louisiana) and have the opportunity to discuss opportunities for graduate or post-baccalaureate studies at The Ohio State University to interested Xavier University of Louisiana students. All expenses associated with this visit will be paid by The Ohio State University.

2. The Ohio State University Graduate Programs Recruiter will attempt to attend each year at least one Graduate and Professional School Day Program conducted at Xavier University of Louisiana; such a visit may be coupled with that described in II.A.I.

### *B. Graduate Student Applicants*

1. Xavier University of Louisiana agrees to disseminate information regarding The Ohio State University's graduate and post-baccalaureate studies to interested students.

2. The Ohio State University agrees to give careful consideration for admission and stipend and fellowship allowance to all qualified students recommended by the Xavier University of Louisiana Dean or faculty.

3. Where deemed appropriate, applicants will be invited to visit The Ohio State University, with the expenses paid in part by The Ohio State University.

## *III. ACADEMIC CHALLENGE UNDERGRADUATE RESEARCH PARTICIPATION PROGRAM (ACURPP)*

1. Xavier University of Louisiana agrees to disseminate information regarding The Ohio State University's ACURPP to interested students.

2. The ACURPP will take under careful consideration for approval those candidates strongly recommended by the Xavier University of Louisiana Dean and will attempt to allocate no fewer than one position annually to such students. In addition to providing such students the usual stipend allowance, an attempt will be made to defray their round-trip travel expenses, locate local housing, and acquaint the student with The Ohio State University Office of Minority Affairs.

## *IV. COORDINATION COMMITTEES*

A joint articulation coordinating committee will be created, having at least two members from each college, and made responsible for all operational aspects of the program. The College of Pharmacy Deans will serve as ex officio members of this committee. This committee will also review the activities described by this agreement and recommend changes for future articulation agreements.

The Xavier University of Louisiana Dean will serve as a consultant to the College of Pharmacy of The Ohio State University on affirmative action activities and as an ex officio member of the Dean's Advisory Committee on Affirmative Action.

# Preparing Minority Pharmacy Students for International Health Service

Rosalyn C. King
Jewel Bazilio Bellegarde

**SUMMARY.** A nine-week internship in international health for a minority pharmacy student is reported. The internship was designed essentially to introduce the student to the WHO concepts of essential drugs and primary health care, to the interaction between primary health care and essential drugs and to explore the role a pharmacist can play in international health.

The internship experience afforded the pharmacy student the opportunity to (1) gather information on the literature of essential drugs and organizations which have programs that relate to essential drugs (2) articulate knowledge gained through the experience and (3) improve his ability to collect, assess and organize information.

This paper describes a nontraditional internship for a Pharmacy student: the International Health and Pharmaceutical Internship of the International Health Institute (IHI) of the Charles R. Drew University of Medicine and Science. The site for the internship was the Institute in Silver Spring, Maryland during the summer of 1990. This nine-week internship was developed in response to the IHI plan to expand the component of its program that related to the provision of essential drugs within its health care delivery projects in developing countries.

---

Rosalyn C. King, Pharm.D., M.P.H., is Director and Jewel Bazilio Bellegarde, M.A., is Training Coordinator at the International Health Institute, Charles R. Drew University of Medicine and Science. Inquires should be addressed to Dr. King at 915 South Belgrade Road, Silver Spring, MD 20902.

The authors acknowledge the background information provided by Linda Uddyback, Program Associate of the Washington Center for Internship and Academic Seminars. Partial support was received from the U.S. Agency for International Development (DAN-5057-G-SS-5091-00).

 

The internship was designed to:

- introduce the student to the World Health Organization and its concepts regarding essential drugs and health care for all;
- permit student interaction with selected health agencies which undertake essential drugs activity within their health care delivery programs;
- enable the student to explore the configuration and interaction between primary health care and international health; and
- provide additional manpower and in the process to broaden the Intern's understanding of the role a pharmacist can play in international health service.

## *INTERNATIONAL HEALTH–POTENTIAL FOR PHARMACIST INVOLVEMENT*

The concept of primary health care has been seen by many member nations of the World Health Organization as a means to achieve an end: *HEALTH CARE FOR ALL BY THE YEAR 2000*. At the International Conference on Primary Health Care held in 1978 in Alma Ata, Russia, a definition of primary health care was proposed by the 134 governments in attendance to include, minimally:

1. education concerning prevailing health problems and methods of preventing and controlling them;
2. promotion of food supply and proper nutrition;
3. an adequate supply of safe water and basic sanitation;
4. maternal and child health care including family planning;
5. immunization against the major infectious diseases;
6. prevention and control of locally endemic diseases;
7. appropriate treatment of common diseases and injuries; and
8. provision of essential drugs (1).

Accordingly, many industrialized countries of the world have some or all these elements of primary health care in their assistance programs to developing countries.

In the United States, it is the Agency for International Development (A.I.D.) which is charged by Congress with providing development assistance from the United States to many countries abroad. The above elements comprise a significant portion of federally funded Health, Population and Nutrition programs abroad. There are, in addition, many private nonprofit or religious groups which provide development assistance as well. However, the achievement of primary health care goals within the context of privately or publicly funded development assistance programs often requires the integration of several components of health care delivery. The provision of essential drugs is the basis of the pharmaceutical segment of primary health care delivery and this segment is essential to the therapeutic, financial and management success of many such health programs.

Many strategies are now developing which concentrate on the ways in which the pharmaceutical component of health service programs in developing countries can be strengthened. These strategies include:

- focusing on essential drugs (i.e., those basic drugs that are used within primary health care to address the main health problems of a community or country);
- increasing the cost-effectiveness and efficiency of drug procurement and use in health programs;
- expanding the supply and appropriate use of essential drugs to the community level through efficient program planning and management;
- indirectly improving the quantity and quality of pharmaceutical sector infrastructure resources; and
- increasing biomedical research in the pharmaceutical sciences within the context of developing country needs.

In all of these strategies, pharmacists can play a useful, exciting and mutually productive role. However, the content of international health as a discipline worthy of career objectives is not usually taught in our Schools of Pharmacy. For these reasons and others mentioned below, it seemed appropriate to initiate the consideration and exploration of international health as a career pathway.

An experience in international health assistance can:

- broaden a pharmacist's understandings of other countries and cultures as the world becomes a global village;
- provide an understanding of the issues in health care delivery services which must be faced by foreign student peers when they return home;

- yield an interesting comparison and contrast between health care delivery, internationally and domestically; and
- demonstrate additional ways a pharmacist can use his/her knowledge system.

## PARTICULAR IMPLICATIONS FOR MINORITY STUDENTS

Minority students of today need to prepare for leadership tomorrow. According to population projections based on the U.S. Census of 1980, the United States, in the 2050s, could become a country in which minorities will approach half of the population (2). As minorities approach this new level, it would be useful if each minority group (and all Americans) could have a broader understanding of the context and cultures from which each "people group" come and of the health issues they bring. One way to obtain this understanding is to participate in development assistance activities abroad.

Further, minority students should be preparing to be represented in the resource pool from which A.I.D. and private groups will draw. The number of pharmacists in international health is small and it is likely that the number of minority pharmacists is minuscule. A survey of organizations and others who hire and train U.S. health professionals for work abroad identified less than 1% of working international health professionals as pharmacists (3). Minority students could make their professional contribution here as well as in other fields of endeavor within the profession of pharmacy. To this end, a mechanism to initiate consideration of international health service as a potential recipient of pharmacist knowledge and skills appeared to be in order.

## COOPERATING ORGANIZATIONS

The internship was structured as a program of the International Health Institute of the Charles R. Drew University of Medicine and Science in which the Institute served as a cooperating agency with the Washington Center for Internships and Academic Seminars. Drew, whose main campus is in Los Angeles, California, is composed of a School of Medicine and a School of Allied Health and has as its mission:

> to conduct medical education and research in the context of service to a defined population and to train persons to provide care with

competence and compassion to this and other underserved populations. (4)

Its School of Medicine is the only historically Black medical school west of the Mississippi River and is also one of the four predominantly Black medical schools in the United States.

The International Health Institute is the operational unit of the University which has the objective of implementing the mission of the University with respect to international service. Location of the Institute in the Metropolitan Washington area is a factor which facilitates the accomplishment of that objective. The part of Institute programming related to pharmaceuticals included, primarily, technical assistance within projects in support of structuring and implementing a drug supply system for the provision of essential drugs to rural communities as well as the implementation of a twelve week course to train health professionals from developing countries in selected aspects of pharmaceutical supply.

Since 1989, the International Health Institute has been privileged to serve as a cooperating agency and host for four Fellows of the Minority Leaders Fellowship Program during the experiential portion of the program as designed by the Washington Center. The Center is an organization which provides internship opportunities around the Metropolitan Washington area for college students. The Washington Center, founded in 1975, is the "largest independent, non-profit organization that enables students to earn college credit for internships and academic seminars in the Nation's capital" (5). Though the Center strives for at least 20% minority participation in its regular Summer Internship Programs, the Minority Leaders Fellowship Program was created and designed specifically for minority college students with the goals of:

- reversing the current trends among young minority men and women by encouraging them to complete their college educations, and
- preparing them to take leading roles in their schools, their communities and the nation at large.

To be accepted as a Fellow, a student must be nominated by their college, be a citizen of the United States, be a member of a minority group (African-American, Asian-American, Hispanic, Native-American, or Pacific Islander), be enrolled in a two- or four-year accredited institution of higher learning and be in good academic standing. Students who have demonstrated initiative and who were active in their community are especially encouraged to apply.

Applications must survive the rigorous scrutiny of a blue-ribbon panel of academic and professional leaders. Applications are scored for academic achievement, communication and analytical skills, demonstrated leadership or initiative and sense of purpose. Those applications with high scores are accepted. Fellows must then be sponsored by a corporate donor who will cover program and housing fees and a cooperating agency which will provide a practical experience and a stipend. The Center is responsible for matching the students with corporate donors and agencies. Of some 400 applications received in 1990, the Minority Fellows Program chose 57 applicants and this group was approximately 11% of the total number of students in programs of the Washington Center.

At Drew/IHI, a Fellow worked on research for a course geared to professionals from the developing world. Two Fellows researched issues in urban health both nationally and internationally. And, one Fellow explored the ways a Pharmacist can use his/her skills within the context of primary health care in the international setting.

## *INTERN SELECTION*

IHI selected the only pharmacy student in the Washington Center program for this experience. However, we did review his background as presented by the Washington Center prior to his arrival at the Institute. The Pharmacy student selected was one of three minority student Interns who were hosted during the Summer of 1990 by the International Health Institute.

The person chosen was of Asian descent and a Junior from the St. John's University College of Pharmacy and Allied Health Professions. He was the first from St. John's and the first from its College of Pharmacy to be included in the program. The student was also the first Pharmacy student to be enrolled in the Minority Leaders Fellowship Program at the Washington Center.

Prior to the arrival of the Intern, IHI had made a decision to consider the expansion of its program efforts that related to the provision of pharmaceuticals within the international health, developing country arena. In order to expand, basic information was needed to assist in targeting opportunities and prioritizing our response. IHI wished to conduct inquiries of other agencies which had program efforts related to essential drugs. The inquiries to be made would require some understanding of the concept of essential drugs as promoted by the World Health Organization and the role of the pharmacist in primary health care.

## *THE INTERNSHIP EXPERIENCE*

The internship experience was organized and managed in three segments: orientation, implementation and evaluation. During the first weeks of his program, the Intern was oriented to Washington, to the Center and to his program. At Drew, a one-day orientation consisted of an introduction to the University's philosophy, goals and purpose; to the IHI staff, the resource center and other logistical and administrative arrangements. The Intern was introduced to the literature resources on essential drugs and viewed a videotape produced by UNICEF (United Nations Children's Fund) on the topic. A major portion of the day was spent on reviewing the work the Intern was expected to accomplish along with the desired output. The Intern was expected to:

1. Update IHI literature resources on a range of topics related to essential drugs;
2. Make telephone calls or conduct visits to selected organizations in order to:

   a. identify individuals involved in program efforts associated with the provision of drugs in developing countries and describe their efforts;
   b. obtain written or other material produced by the organization visited;

3. With assistance, update IHI's data bank by including suitable pharmacy-related questions on the consultant registry forms;
4. Meet with the Director or her designee as requested;
5. Compile the following information into a report:

   a. an annotated bibliography of materials collected during the internship;
   b. a list of all organizations contacted along with key contacts, their title and a description of their efforts;
   c. a mailing list of Schools of Pharmacy worldwide and Pharmacy associations within the United States; and
   d. other documents produced during the internship.

In general, the Intern was expected to apply and articulate knowledge gained through the educational experience as well as improve his/her ability to collect, assess and organize information.

At the beginning of June, Fellows arrived in Washington for an intensive, ten-week educational program which was both theoretical and experiential, and which exposed him/her to national leaders in many sectors. The theoretical component, one week, preceded the nine-week experience and began with a seminar on leadership theory and skill development. This component continued with nine, weekly seminars which encouraged each participant to develop and recognize his leadership style as well as to discuss the history and culture of minorities in America.

The experiential component consisted of a nine-week, full-time internship at Drew/IHI, which was the cooperating agency. During the first two weeks of his internship at IHI, the Fellow developed, in conjunction with the Institute's Director and Training Coordinator, a Learning Contract which incorporated all of the elements of the detailed scope of work he received from Drew as well as personal objectives which he set for himself. The Intern was also encouraged to attend evening and breakfast lecture/speaker series sponsored by the Center. He was required to participate in an academic course (offered by the Center) one evening per week during the entire ten-week period. The Pharmacy student chose to take a Public Speaking course.

One of the unplanned experiences during the internship was the Intern's attendance at the National Council for International Health annual conference. Several sessions and workshops dealt with issues associated with the provision of essential drugs to populations in developing countries.

The internship experience was managed by the Director of the Institute, a public health pharmacist. The Training Coordinator maintained day-to-day supervision. The Fellow was given desk space within IHI offices and participated in staff meetings. General personal/logistical support, however, was managed by the Center. This included housing and other backing such as career planning service, guidance and counseling. These were available, as needed, from the Center through a staff liaison who organized student life activities, tours and field trips.

## *INTERNSHIP EVALUATION*

There were three assessments during the internship. The first was the development of a learning contract which outlined the goals, objectives and ground rules of the internship. This exercise gave an early indication of the Fellow's assimilation of the content of the concepts emanating from the orientation and early discussions at Drew/IHI. The student documented his understanding of Drew as a University and IHI as one of its components, listed the substantive knowledge he would gain from the experience, indicated the duties he would perform while at IHI and who would supervise and evaluate his performance. This contract was agreed upon by the Fellow, Drew and the Center.

A mid-point evaluation, designed to review the Intern's progress in fulfilling the learning contract, was carried out using a structured format. The areas examined were the internship environment at Drew/IHI, the general growth of the intern and the perceived increase in his level of skills and application of knowledge. In each area, the rater, on a scale of 1 to 5, specified whether or not there was improvement needed (scale of 1), progress was satisfactory or progress exceeded expectations (scale of 5). The evaluator could also make general comments regarding productivity.

There were three parts to the final evaluation: the Drew/IHI evaluation, the site visit of the Faculty Advisor who served as the Dean of St. John's University College of Pharmacy and Allied Health Professions and the overall evaluation by the Washington Center. Drew/IHI Fellows were required to make an oral presentation to the staff of the Institute and to submit a report along with supporting documentation as detailed in the original scope of work. Drew combined the site visit of the Dean with the requirement for an oral presentation. Drew's ending assessment centered largely on the extent to which the goals and objectives, as detailed by the student in his learning contract and by Drew in the scope of work, were documented and achieved. The Director of the Institute was asked by the Washington Center to recommend a grade to the Intern's faculty advisor.

## *CONCLUSION*

It was evident that the Fellow had a positive view of the total experience. He stated in his departing reflections that "I have gained a greater understanding of Pharmacy and International Health. It is hard to consider that three-fourths of the world's population belong to the developing world yet international health is considered a small field in the health care professions" (6).

There has been an important introduction and exposure to ways in which he can use his professional skills to serve, if he wishes, with competence and compassion, to underserved populations wherever they may be. International service can now be viewed as a viable career option. This view can be shared by the Intern with his peers and others within his educational and community environment as he moves to continue his leadership role.

Having hosted the Minority Leaders Fellowship Program over the past two years, The Charles R. Drew University of Medicine and Science is further along in expanding the pool of minority leaders who serve the underserved wherever they are encountered. Unfortunately, plans for program expansion using the data derived from the internship were curtailed due to a lack of funding. It may be continued once adequate funding is identified.

It is hoped that this paper serves to nudge the profession of Pharmacy to take a closer look at International health as a potential career option for pharmacy graduates whose personal and professional interests meet at the juncture of the professions of pharmacy and public health.

## REFERENCES

1. World Health Organization. Alma Ata 1978-Primary health care. Geneva, Switzerland: World Health Organization, 1978.

2. Spencer G. Projections of the Hispanic population 1983-2080 in Bureau of Census current population reports. Washington, DC: U.S. Bureau of Census, 1986. Series P-25, No. 995. November 1986.

3. Baker TD, Weisman C, Piwoz E. U.S. health professionals in international health. Am J Public Health 1984; 74:438-41.

4. Drew/UCLA Medical Education Program. Los Angeles, CA: Charles R. Drew University of Medicine and Science, 1989.

5. Minority Leaders 1990 Fellowship Program. Washington, DC: Washington Center for Internships and Academic Seminars, 1990.

6. Kennedy T. Presentation to the staff of the International Health Institute. August 3, 199

# An Educational Pipeline into Pharmacy for Minority Students

J. W. Carmichael, Jr.
Sr. Joanne Bauer
Jacqueline T. Hunter
Deidre D. Labat
J. Ann Privett
John P. Sevenair

**SUMMARY.** During the past fifteen years Xavier University of Louisiana (XU) has grown to become #1 nationally in placing African Americans into pharmacy (and #2 in placing African Americans into medicine). While many factors have contributed to this success, one of the most visible is the "educational pathway" developed by Arts & Sciences faculty to motivate and prepare African Americans for entry into pharmacy, medicine, and similar health professions. This pathway currently includes science-related summer programs for students every year beginning in junior high

J. W. Carmichael, Jr., Ph.D., is Professor of Chemistry, Sr. Joanne Bauer, S.B.S., Ph.D., is Assistant Professor of Chemistry, Jacqueline T. Hunter, Ph.D., is Professor of Biology, Deidre D. Labat, Ph.D., is Professor of Biology, J. Ann Privett is Assistant Professor of Chemistry, and John P. Sevenair, Ph.D., is Professor of Chemistry, all at Xavier University of Louisiana, New Orleans, LA 70125.

 

and continuing until entry into college, as well as extensive revision of Xavier's entry-level science and mathematics courses including almost all of those required in the prepharmacy curriculum, so as to promote student success.

## INTRODUCTION

Over the past fifteen years, a period during which the number of students entering college interested in science-related careers was decreasing nationwide, Xavier University of Louisiana (XU) more than doubled the number of students it placed into health professions schools from an average of 43/year in the mid-70s to over 100/year over the past three year period. Of even greater importance, more than 90% of the XU students who gained entry into health professions school over this period were African Americans, a group whose severe underrepresentation in the health professions adversely affects the health care received by African Americans. Over the past three-year period, Xavier was #1 nationally in placing African Americans into schools of pharmacy and #2 in the nation in placing African Americans into medical school.

Xavier's success in preparing African Americans for entry into pharmacy is the result of a number of factors, many of which are described elsewhere in this publication. The purpose of this article, however, is to describe efforts in Xavier's College of Arts and Sciences to recruit and prepare African Americans (including prepharmacy students) for a broad spectrum of the health professions.

Xavier University of Louisiana is a historically Black Catholic institution whose enrollment in the fall of 1990 was slightly less than 3,000–an increase of one-third from five years ago. The primary focus of Xavier's undergraduate programs is the liberal arts. Natural science majors in the College of Arts and Sciences are required to take 45 semester hours of courses outside the sciences, the majority of which are in the humanities (including languages, literature, history, philosophy, and theology). The distribution of Xavier's undergraduates by major, however, is very unusual for a liberal arts institution. In the fall of 1990, 23% of the University's undergraduates were enrolled in prepharmacy or pharmacy, and another 23% were enrolled in chemistry or biology. Most of the latter are interested in medicine or dentistry. Substantial enrollments in engineering, computer science, and related disciplines gave the sciences at Xavier approximately 50% of the student body.

## *SOME REASONS FOR XAVIER'S SUCCESS*

Xavier is a small institution with meager financial resources located in a state not noted for educational achievement. In spite of these limitations, XU has had much greater success in preparing African-American youth for entry into the highly competitive health professions than more affluent colleges and universities. Research has shown that Xavier's success is not the result of recruitment alone. While Xavier is not an open admissions institution, it also does not accept only the cream of African-American high school graduates. In the recent past, freshmen entering Xavier have had an average high school grade point average of 2.80 and an average ACT score (old scores, not the "enhanced" test given since the fall of 1989) of approximately 16. This ACT score is approximately equivalent to a combined SAT score of 760. Instead, Xavier's success is a direct result of the various activities implemented by the University to increase the probability that African-American students will succeed in the health professions.

This is illustrated by comparing the percentage of African-American freshmen who succeed at Xavier versus those who succeed nationally. A recent ETS study indicates that only 24% of high ability African-Americans (defined to be the top 2% of ACT/SAT scores) who enter four-year colleges complete a degree program and gain entry into any graduate or professional school (1). Studies at Xavier indicate that 40% of those with ACT scores from 12 to 17, 49% of those with scores of 18 to 23, and 80% of students with scores of 24 and above completed the Prepharmacy program and gained entry into Pharmacy (2). These results have been verified by a similar study of Xavier's premedical program (3).

Much of Xavier's success in placing African Americans into pharmacy is the direct result of careful implementation and continuing improvement of programs developed by the University's science and mathematics faculty (within the College of Arts and Sciences). These programs are effective because, taken together they form an educational pipeline which identifies students with potential and interest early, and provides encouragement and academic enrichment on an ongoing basis until completion of sophomore-level mathematics and science courses. In retrospect, this pipeline appears to have been designed rigorously from first principles and as a result of extensive planning (4). However, it is important to note that instead it developed as science and mathematics faculty attempted to address problems, one at a time, starting from the critical transition from high school to college, and then proceeding on to address other problems as time permitted (and sometimes when it didn't). This "educational pipeline" is described below.

## THE SUMMER SCIENCE ACADEMY

The primary focus of Xavier's science-related activities for precollege students is a series of four summer enrichment programs designed to prepare students for the major mathematics or science courses they will take during their freshman and sophomore (Prepharmacy) years. These programs are known collectively as the Summer Science Academy. The specific programs are:

- MathStar, a two-week summer program that prepares students for algebra courses, usually the first rigorous math course they encounter. Students usually enroll during the summer between the 8th and 9th grades.
- BioStar, a three-week summer program that prepares students for high school biology. Students typically attend during the summer between the 9th and 10th grades.
- ChemStar, a three-week summer program that prepares students for high school chemistry (4-6). Students usually attend the ChemStar program in the summer between their 10th and 11th grades.
- SOAR (Stress On Analytical Reasoning), a four-week, problem-solving based high school/college bridge program (4,7,8). Students attend the program following either their junior or senior year in high school. Those who complete the SOAR program after their junior year may enter Xavier during the summer after their senior year under a newly developed program that gives them a head start on their college requirements.

Xavier's precollege summer programs were developed one at a time by mathematics and science faculty over the past fifteen years. Experience gained from previous development was used when proceeding to new endeavors, as was the expertise of dedicated teachers from a variety of local schools. Although the four programs in Xavier's Summer Science Academy differ in response to content demands and the educational level of the participants, all contain the following features to some degree:

- *Integration of problem-solving with content.*
- *At least two hours of homework daily.*
- *Daily quizzes which test the previous day's work.*
- *Rapid grading* so students can use past performance to help prepare for the future quizzes.
- *Emphasis on vocabulary and/or reading skills.*
- *Group competitions* designed to promote the formation of peer support groups based on academics.
- *The use of successful Xavier students as role models.* These students serve as group leaders. Each organizes a group of students for competitions, inspires by example, calls all who are tardy or absent, and generally serves as an older brother or sister for the summer program participants.
- *Parental involvement.* Parents are invited with participants to an opening ceremony and orientation the day before the beginning of each program, and are sent report cards at least once per week. Parents are also invited to an awards ceremony at the end of the programs at which all students receive graduation certificates and are given the opportunity to show their parents what they have achieved.
- *Social activities* which let the program participants see that students who succeed in the sciences are not necessarily nerds. These include pizza parties, dances, and (for older students) a walking tour of the French Quarter.

The success of the programs is indicated by the fact that 1,260 students applied to the programs in 1990, and funds were available to accept 643 students into the programs. Over 99% of the participants were African-Americans; 82% were female.

## *THE MODIFICATION OF ENTRY-LEVEL MATH AND SCIENCE COURSES TO SUPPORT THE UNDERPREPARED*

Xavier's Arts and Sciences programs identify and encourage students capable of succeeding in pharmacy and other science based professions are not limited to the precollege years. The mathematics and science departments have taken equally unorthodox approaches to their entry-level courses (4). These courses are not viewed as filters designed to eliminate the underprepared as they are at many other institutions. Key entry-level courses including general biology, general chemistry, organic chemistry, general physics, and precalculus, have been modified to provide extensive support for the underprepared while maintaining high standards (9-11).

The most basic change in the entry-level science courses was the adoption of the philosophy that course content, teaching methodology, and rate of presentation should be determined by the relevant department as a whole, and not by individual lecturers or textbooks. This standardization not only made it possible to improve support for the underprepared (for example, tutors know exactly what is covered in all lecture sections of a course), but also provided a strong support mechanism for part-time or new faculty. The system is sustained by a series of workbooks which tell the student exactly what he/she is to learn, where additional information about the topic may be found, and sample problems selected for their importance by faculty who actually teach the courses. Although the content of the workbook is determined by the department as a whole, it is not static. Workbooks are rewritten and revised frequently, responding to departmental decisions to stress different areas or to the development of new and better ways of teaching.

One or more of these key mathematics and science courses have other unusual features which contribute significantly to the University's success in placing African-Americans into Pharmacy and other areas in the health professions, as follows . . .

- *Inquiry-based laboratory experiments* require students to "do science." That is, they collect data, analyze it, and make predictions based on that analysis, rather than merely verifying something already known in cookbook fashion (12-14).
- *Special exercises help students improve their test-taking skills.* Students in general chemistry, and to some extent in general biology, are repeatedly required to work sections from the quantitative or reading sections of published examinations used to judge the qualifications of students wishing to gain entry to graduate or health professional schools.
- *Systematic efforts throughout the freshman and sophomore years improve general, not scientific, vocabulary.* Students enrolled in general biology, general chemistry, organic chemistry, and physics must study from 40-80 general vocabulary words weekly. They receive points in each course for performance on short quizzes that check their mastery of the words. The vocabulary words are divided

into two sets, each of which is covered twice. The first set is used in general biology and general chemistry, the second in organic chemistry and general physics.

- *Systematic efforts help students learn to visualize in three dimensions.* Students in general chemistry, general biology, organic chemistry, and physics are all required to build appropriate physical models repeatedly, in an effort to improve their ability to visualize physical objects in three dimensions. This ability has been found to be related to the ability to perform well in many science courses.
- *A systematic effort is made during the freshman year to get students in general chemistry and biology to form study groups.* Members of these groups are expected to work together for the good of all. Students who do not perform up to expectations are advised individually to form study groups. In addition, effort is devoted to helping them find an appropriate study group. In some instances, study groups are formed by hiring a student who is doing well in the course to serve as a study group coordinator.

## *OTHER SUPPORT FOR THE UNDERGRADUATE STUDENT*

Additional factors contribute to Xavier's success in preparing African-American youth for entry into the highly competitive biomedical sciences.

- *Most students entering Xavier declare a major when matriculating.* Prepharmacy students are immediately assigned an academic advisor in the College of Pharmacy. Close advisor-student interaction is both encouraged and expected at Xavier. In order to ensure that it really exists, all students enrolled in freshman biology and freshman chemistry receive points in both courses for keeping an up-to-date record of their grades on an "advisor's card" signed weekly by their academic advisor.
- *Xavier's science departments provide extensive tutoring for students in entry-level science courses.* The departments of Biology, Chemistry, Mathematics, and Physics all operate tutorial services designed to help students enrolled in the entry-level courses in their respective departments. Providing effective tutorial services is relatively easy in these courses because the courses are "standardized" as discussed above. The tutors in all of the services are upper-level students who performed well in the courses the previous year. They

know exactly what was covered, how problems were worked, and how the present topic is related to past ones. As a result it is relatively easy to prepare tutors for their jobs. Because the tutors are able to provide assistance directly coordinated to the courses for which they tutor, students are more willing to seek their assistance.

- *The faculty most concerned with the above efforts have voluntarily organized as the Science Education Research Group (SERG).* This group meets weekly to plan and administer the programs discussed above (14). Perhaps even more importantly, the SERG provides support for the faculty involved. So far they have managed to avoid, or at least minimize, one of the most common reasons why successful educational innovations are terminated–burnout.

Evaluation has provided two clear types of evidence that Xavier's modified entry-level science courses are more effective than traditional courses. First, more students pass the science courses at present than passed before the courses were modified. For instance, the percentage who pass freshman-level courses in biology and chemistry with a "C" or higher has increased from approximately 40% before modification to 60% or so at present. Second, those who are passing these courses now are also scoring higher (on the average) on comparable final exams and/or appropriate standardized exams than did their counterparts before the courses were modified.

Although there is extensive support in the freshman-level biology and chemistry courses at Xavier, this support is purposely decreased at the sophomore level so that the students can perform at a competitive level without "crutches" when they enter the College of Pharmacy.

## ACKNOWLEDGMENTS

We gratefully acknowledge financial support from the following sources for activities as indicated:

- *The Health Careers Opportunity Program (HCOP), Division of Disadvantaged Assistance, Bureau of Health Professions, HHS*, for funds to develop the nontraditional activities (vocabulary-building, improving ability to visualize in 3-D, etc.) in XU's entry-level science courses which, after field-testing, were integrated into the courses so that no external funding is required to maintain them and support students in SOAR, the University's high school/college bridge program.

- *The Howard Hughes Medical Institute* for funds to further modify and better integrate the summer programs, to upgrade basic laboratories, and to support students in all four of the University's science-related precollege summer programs–MathStar, BioStar, ChemStar, and SOAR.

## REFERENCES

1. Hilton TL, Schrader WB. Pathways to graduate school: an empirical study based on national longitudinal data. GRE No. 82-21. Educational Testing Service, 1985.

2. Grace M, Carmichael JW Jr, Hunter JT, Labat DD, Sevenair JP. Assessment of the ability of a prepharmacy program to serve Black Americans. J Natl Pharm Assoc 1989; 33(1):23-9.

3. Carmichael JW Jr, Bauer J, Hunter JT, Labat DD, Sevenair JP. An assessment of a premedical program in terms of its ability to serve Black Americans. J Natl Med Assoc 1988; 80:1094-104.

4. Carmichael JW Jr, Hunter JT, Labat DD, Sevenair JP, Bauer J. An educational pathway into biology-and chemistry-based careers for Black Americans. J Coll Sci Teach 1988; 17:370-4.

5. Sevenair JP, Carmichael JW Jr. A high school chemistry prep course designed by college faculty to increase the number of Black Americans in science related careers. J Coll Sci Teach 1988; 18:51-4.

6. Sevenair JP, Carmichael JW Jr, Bauer J, McLean M. ChemStar student manual. 2nd ed. Champaign, IL: Stipes Publishing Co., 1989.

7. Whimbey A, Carmichael JW Jr, Jones LW, Hunter JT, Vincent HA. Teaching critical reading and analytical reasoning in Project SOAR. J Read 1980; 24(1):5-9.

8. Carmichael JW Jr, Hunter JT, Jones LW, Ryan MA, Sevenair JP, Vincent HA. Project SOAR (Stress On Analytical Reasoning). 2nd ed. Instructor's manual for Project SOAR (Stress On Analytical Reasoning). 2nd ed. Champaign, IL: Stipes Publishing Co., 1989.

9. Carmichael JW Jr, Bauer J, Sevenair JP, Robinson D. First-year chemistry with built-in support for the underprepared. Int Newsl Chem Educ 1985; (23)15.

10. Bauer J, Carmichael JW Jr. General chemistry handbook–a student manual for success in first-year chemistry. 3rd ed. Champaign, IL: Stipes Publishing, 1989.

11. Sevenair JP, O'Connor SE, Nazery M. A nontraditional organic chemistry course. J Coll Sci Teach 1989; 18:236-9.

12. Ryan MA, Carmichael JW Jr. A Piagetian-based general chemistry laboratory sequence for science majors. J Chem Educ 1980; 57:642-5.

13. Bauer J, Allen LR, Carmichael JW Jr, Ryan MA, Robinson DK, Sevenair JP, Wells BK. General chemistry laboratory manual. 3rd ed. Champaign, IL: Stipes Publishing Co., 1989.

14. Sevenair JP, Carmichael JW Jr, Bauer J, Hunter JT, Labat D, Vincent H, Jones LW. SERG: a model for colleges without graduate programs. J Coll Sci Teach 1987; 16:444-6

# Florida A&M University: Impact of Private and Federal Funding on the Development of Graduate Pharmaceutical Education and Research

Johnnie L. Early, II
Kinfe K. Redda
Pauline Hicks
Magdi Soliman
Karam Soliman
Larry D. Fannin
Walter L. Smith
Charles U. Smith
Henry Lewis, III
Lambros P. Tterlikkis
Farid Stino
Thomas Fitzgerald
Frederick S. Humphries
Charles A. Walker
Israel Tribble
Richard A. Hogg
Gertrude L. Simmons
Leedell W. Neyland

Johnnie L. Early, II, Ph.D., is Dean and Professor, Kinfe K. Redda, Ph.D., is Professor, Pauline Hicks, AMD, is University Librarian, Magdi Soliman, Ph.D., is Professor, Karam Soliman, Ph.D., is Professor, Larry D. Fannin, Pharm.D., is Associate Professor, Walter L. Smith, Ph.D., is Director and Professor, Charles U. Smith, Ph.D., is Dean of Graduate Studies and Distinguished Professor of Sociology, all at Florida A&M University, Tallahassee, Fl 32307. Henry Lewis, III Pharm. D., is Dean at the Texas Southern University College of Pharmacy and Health Sciences, 3100 Cleburne Street, Houston, TX 77004. Lambros P. Tterlikkis, Ph.D., is Professor, Farid Stino, Ph.D., is Statistician, Thomas Fitzgerald, Ph.D., is Professor, Frederick S. Humphries, Ph.D., is President, all at Florida A&M University, Tallahassee, FL 32307. Charles A. Walker, Ph.D., is Special Expert at the NIH National Library of Medicine, 8600 Rockville Pike, Bethesda, MD 20894. Israel Tribble, Ed.D., is President, Florida Endowment Fund, 201 E. Kennedy Bldg., Suite 1525, Tampa, FL 33602. Richard A. Hogg, Ph.D., is Provost and Vice President, Gertrude L. Simmons, Ph.D., is Former Vice President, and Leedell W. Neyland, Ph.D., is Professor, all at Florida A&M University, Tallahassee, FL 32307.

 

**SUMMARY.** Federal, state, and private funding laid the foundation for both graduate pharmaceutical education and research in the Florida A&M University College of Pharmacy and Pharmaceutical Sciences. Initial (1973) Minority Biomedical Research Support Program funding led to the 1976 establishment of the M.S. program in pharmacology/toxicology. The MBRS program's maturation included the implementation of presubmission review procedures for grant proposals which yielded significant improvement in proposal competitiveness. From 1980 to 1984, the MBRS grant increased from six investigators to 12, and a 250% increase in funding. M.S. program success led to the Ph.D. program in pharmaceutical sciences (pharmacology/toxicology, medicinal chemistry, pharmaceutics, and pharmacy administration) in 1985. The 59 other pharmacy schools with graduate programs produced 13 African Americans with Ph.D. degrees from 1984-89. Florida A&M University graduated 5 in April 1991 to become America's preeminent provider of such personnel. Three of the 5 were McKnight Fellows; all were supported by both MBRS and RCMI. Funds provided by the Centers for Disease Control/Agency for Toxic Substances and Disease Registry cooperative agreement with the Association of Minority Health Professions Schools led to implementation of a Ph.D. track in environmental toxicology in 1990. Federal and corporate funding assists graduate student support, and helped establish an endowed chair. The College successfully competed for a Research Centers at Minority Institutions grant in 1985 which has sparked an increase in refereed publications from 19/year in 1983-87, to 36 in 1989, an 89% increase. Five proposals were submitted in 1983, compared to 30 funded grants in 1990. Grant support increased from $600,000 in 1983 to $3.7 million in 1990. The College is now 11th among pharmacy schools in NIH ($1.7 million) funding. The quality of library services and laboratory animal facilities has been enhanced.

## *INTRODUCTION*

Historically Black or African American Colleges and Universities (HBCUs) have traditionally trained a disproportionately large number of the professionals who provide health care for underserved communities, and students who subsequently earn advanced degrees. The objective of this paper is to report on the impact of private and federal funding on the development of graduate pharmaceutical education and research in the Florida Agricultural and Mechanical University (FAMU) College of Pharmacy and Pharmaceutical Sciences, the only Historically African American unit of the nine member State University System of Florida.

The Minority Biomedical Research Support (MBRS) Program provided the essential funding of $23,000 in 1973 to begin research in the College. This funding laid the foundation for both research, and the graduate program which began in 1976 with the M.S. program in pharmacology/toxicology. The MBRS program reached a significant level in 1984, during the efforts of the College to win approval for the Ph.D. degree program in pharmaceutical sciences. Approval was granted and the first students admitted in January 1985 to the initial track, pharmacology/toxicology, with medicinal chemistry, pharmaceutics, and pharmacy administration approved for the future. While MBRS and R01 supported research yielded significant contributions in several areas, the most notable are the patents of Henry J. Lee, Ph.D., for the highly potent, but less toxic derivatives of prednisolone (U.S. Patent No. 4,588,530, "Anti-inflammatory Prednisolone Steroids," 1986 and U.S. Patent No. 4,762,919, "Anti-inflammatory Carboxy Pregnan Derivatives," 1988).

The College qualified for the Research Centers at Minority Institutions (RCMI) program because of its Doctor of Pharmacy program, which began in January 1978, and the Ph.D. program. The College received the fourth most competitive priority score, and the largest award among the seven initial institutions to receive RCMI funding in 1985. The RCMI awards of both 1985 and 1990 have developed and continue to maintain the infrastructure necessary for a competitive graduate and research program. The impact of RCMI has been significant, measured in terms of the marked increase in the number of refereed publications, and the development of the Clinical Pharmacology Research Unit.

National Aeronautics and Space Administration funding has been realized for both student support, and significant research conducted as part of the Cosmos missions which were launched in 1987 and 1989, on the pineal gland, and ongoing research on stress. As a part of the cooperative agreement between the Association of Minority Health Professions Schools and the Centers for Disease Control and Agency for Toxic Substances and Disease Registry, the College received funding in 1988 to develop environmental toxicology as a track in the graduate program. The Ph.D. program has also attracted funding for students from the Florida Endowment Fund, Delores Auzenne Scholarship, Patricia Roberts-Harris Program, the American Foundation for Pharmaceutical Education, National Aeronautics and Space Administration, and the U.S. Department of Energy.

Pfizer Central Research awarded the first corporate fellowship for a graduate student in 1990; The Procter & Gamble Company, Research and Development Department awarded a second graduate scholarship in 1991. Of universal benefit, is the entry of FAMU as a producer of minorities with the Ph.D. in pharmaceutical sciences. The seven graduates to date have entered postdoctoral training (4), and become employed (3) in academic institutions, with a pharmaceutical manufacturer, and a government agency. The first to complete postdoctoral training is now employed with a pharmaceutical manufacturer.

## *THE FOUNDATIONAL ESSENTIALITY OF THE MBRS PROGRAM*

One of the maturing experiences that grew out of the MBRS program was the need to improve the quality of proposals through a review process prior to submission. In 1980, prior to the implementation of this procedure, an MBRS proposal entitled "Biochemical and Pharmacological Investigations" earned a priority score of 250. Subsequently, the program director organized an internal review by faculty members for a supplemental application. This proposal received a priority score of 219. In 1983, both the internal and external review procedures were employed on the renewal application, "Biochemical and Pharmacological Investigations," which subsequently received a priority score of 198. In that same year, a proposal was developed to host a national scientific meeting, the "Minority Biomedical Research Support Symposium," and it received a winning priority score of 198. A 1984 supplement to the MBRS parent grant received a priority score of 206. In 1985, applications for two proposals: the "Research Centers at Minority Institutions (RCMI), Florida A&M University Research Center," and the "MBRS Thematic Grant Program: Chronopharmacological and Chronotherapeutic Investigations," were reviewed and subsequently received priority scores of 165 and 126, respectively (1).

The internal review involves fellow scientists who critically evaluate and make suggestions on the proposal. These individuals, who may not be active in the same area of research, can make useful observations on the focus, clarity, and completeness of the proposal. In contrast, the external review involves scientists who are devoid of any affiliation with the principal investigator. The College of Pharmacy retains a pool of external reviewers, and its RCMI advisory committee members for this purpose. Investigators have the option of nominating alternate reviewers.

## *MINORITY BIOMEDICAL FUNDING AND RESEARCH TOPICS 1988-92*

FAMU has continued receiving MBRS funding since 1973. The latest NIH/MBRS notice of grant award shows that FAMU received a total of $3.5 million (direct and indirect costs) for the period of March 1989-February 1993 (Table 1). That brings the funding level to an overall total of 11.4 million dollars since 1973. Recipients of the MBRS award were faculty from the College of Pharmacy and Pharmaceutical Sciences as well as the College of Arts and Sciences as shown in Tables 1-5.

The objectives of the current award are to expand and strengthen the capabilities of FAMU investigators in the area of biomedical sciences research, to provide undergraduate students with hands-on experience in the fundamentals of scientific research, and to motivate them to pursue biomedical research careers. It also has the purpose, to train graduate students in the state-of-the-art research in the biomedical sciences with emphasis on pharmacology, toxicology, medicinal chemistry, biochemistry or molecular biology. Tables 2, 3, 4 and 5 provide a detailed accounting of principal investigators, their funding, and research topics for 1984-89, 1981-84, 1978-81 and 1973-78, respectively. Table 6 shows that over the several award periods, 996 students (930 undergraduate and 66 graduate) have received MBRS support. Ninety percent of the students were African American, and 10% were Hispanics and Asian-Americans.

The MBRS support of undergraduate students (Table 7) allows them time to focus on solving a research problem designed to develop their understanding of the science. Most undergraduates present a paper(s) at the annual MBRS Symposium, America's largest gathering of minority scientists, and students. The students also present their research results at other meetings (American Society of Pharmacology and Therapeutics, Society of Toxicology, Federation of American Societies of Experimental Biology, and the American Chemical Society) where they gain valuable experiences and perspectives on research careers. A common experience of undergraduate students is being mistaken for graduate students as a result of their professional handling of both the presentation and resulting questions. It is our assessment that both the presentation and laboratory

Table 1. MBRS Principal Investigators, Funding Level and Research Topics, 1989-1993.

| Principal Investigator | Research Topic | 1989-1993 |
|---|---|---|
| Blyden, G. T | Clinical Pharmacology | $ 211,787 |
| Dhanarajan, Z. C.[a] | Biochemistry | 271,609 |
| Early, II, J. L. | Selenium-Induced Hyperglycemia | 259,898 |
| Fitzgerald, T. J. | Synth. Med. Chem./Colchicine | 316,864 |
| Friedman, R. O.[b] | Biological Sciences | 117,013 |
| Hamilton, F. D.[a] | Biochemistry | 133,251 |
| Lee, H. L. | Synth. Med. Chem./Steroids | 140,551 |
| Ollapally, A. P.[a] | Synth. Org. Chem./Anticancer | 216,799 |
| Redda, K. K. | (Administration Grant) | 271,770 |
| Redda, K. K. | Synth. Med. Chem./N-Heterocyc. | 345,526 |
| Soliman, K. F. | Neuropharmacology/Physiology | 156,892 |
| Soliman, M. I. | Chronopharmacology | 124,770 |
| | Total direct cost: | $2,566,730 |
| | Indirect cost: | 949,673 |
| | Overall Total: | $3,516,403 |

[a]Chemistry department.

[b]Biology department.

skills of an undergraduate student of two years' training are equivalent to those of a first-year graduate student. Moreover, MBRS students are found to be more likely than their non-MBRS counterparts to enter graduate school. Former students are recipients of: doctor of philosophy degrees in pharmacokinetics, pharmacology/toxicology, and biochemistry; doctor of medicine and of professional pharmacy degrees. Several are enrolled in similar programs.

The Research Apprentice Programs of NIH and NSF have served as

Table 2. MBRS Principal Investigator, Funding Level, and Research Topics, 1984-1989.

| Principal Investigator | Research Topic | 1984-1989 |
|---|---|---|
| Bradshaw, W. G. | Clinical Psychologist | $ 90,730 |
| Cottrell, P. T.[a] | Physical Chem./Electroxidation | 167,663 |
| Early,II, J. L.(84-88) | MBRS Administrative Grant | 221,180 |
| Early,II, J. L. | Pharmacology/Toxico. Selenium | 396,611 |
| Early,II, J. L.(1985) | National MBRS Symposium | 122,998 |
| Early,II, J. L. (1986) | National MBRS Symposium | 139,295 |
| Early,II, J. L.(1987-88) | Student Income Supplement | 13,207 |
| Fitzgerald, T. J. | Synthetic Med. Chem./ Colchicine | 205,999 |
| Holder, M. S. | Cardiovascular Physiology | 35,554 |
| Lamba, S. S. | Synthetic/National Prod. Chem. | 72,219 |
| Lee, H. J. | Synthetic Med. Chem./ Steroids | 168,857 |
| Ollapally, A. P.[a] | Synthetic Org. Chem./ Anti-Cancer | 366,861 |
| Parker, V. D. | Clinical Pharmacology | 71,060 |
| Redda, K. K. | Synthetic Med. Chem./ N-Heterocycles | 186,256 |
| Redda, K. K. (1988-89) | MBRS Administrative Grant | 37,060 |
| Redda, K. K. (1989) | Student Income Supplement | 72,382 |
| Soliman, K. F. | Neuropharmacology/ Physiology | 144,035 |
| Soliman, M. I. | Instrument Grant | 25,000 |
| Tterlikkis, L. P. | Physical/Biol. Chem. | 264,092 |
| Walker, C. A. | Chronopharmacology | 83,840 |
| | Total Direct Cost | $2,884,899 |
| | Indirect Cost | 786,135 |
| | Overall Total | $3,671,034 |

[a]Chemistry department.

Table 3. MBRS Principal Investigator, Funding Level, and Research Topics, 1981-1984.

| Principal Investigator | Research Topic | 1981-84 |
|---|---|---|
| Day, J. L. | Medicinal Chemistry/Anti-cancer | $ 158,685 |
| Early,II, J. L. | MBRS Administration Grant | 251,374 |
| Early,II, J. L. | Toxicology/Selenium | 190,023 |
| Fitzgerald, T. J. | Synthetic Med. Chem/Colchicine | 100,792 |
| Holder, M. S. | Cardiovascular Physiology | 106,840 |
| Lee, H. J. | Synthetic Med. Chemistry/Steriods | 128,002 |
| Lewis, B. A. | Microbiology | 46,648 |
| Nwangwu, P. | Medicinal Chemistry | 38,006 |
| Ollapally, A. P. | Synth. Organic Chem./Anti-Cancer | 138,333 |
| Shetty, A. S.[b] | Biological Sciences | 147,293 |
| Soliman, K. F. | Chornopharmacology/Physiology | 82,012 |
| Turner, R. W.[a] | Organic Chemistry | 167,226 |
| | Total Direct Cost | $1,555,234 |
| | Indirect Cost | 588,596 |
| | Overall Total | $2,143,830 |

[a]Chemistry department.

[b]Biology department.

linkages for the MBRS program. Since 1982, the College of Pharmacy offered opportunities for summer research to FAMU Developmental Research School and other high school students in the Research Apprentice Program funded by either NIH, Division of National Institute of General Medical Sciences, or National Science Foundation. Federal funding is supplemented by institutional funds to allow greater student participation. Ten participants have entered the College of Pharmacy, and 5 have graduated. Several others have matriculated in the natural sciences

Table 4. MBRS Principal Investigator, Funding Level, and Research Topics, 1978-1981.

| Principal Investigator | Research Topic | 1978-81 |
|---|---|---|
| Early,II, J. L. | MBRS Administration Grant | $ 45,577 |
| Early,II, J. L. | Toxicology/Selenium | 35,850 |
| Ikediobi, C.[a] | Biochemistry | 41,441 |
| Ollapally, A. P.[a] | Synth. Organic Chem./Anti-Cancer | 111,748 |
| Lee, H. J. | Synthetic Med. Chemistry/Steriods | 128,002 |
| Shetty, A. S.[b] | Biochemistry | 105,515 |
| Tterlikkis, L. P. | Administration Grant | 91,084 |
| Tterlikkis, L. P. | Pharmaceutics | 234,260 |
| | Total Direct Cost | $ 805,734 |
| | Indirect Cost | 322,299 |
| | Overall Total | $1,128,028 |

[a]Chemistry department.

[b]Biology department.

and engineering at FAMU, and other institutions. To date, Leonard K. Holt, is currently a Ph.D. candidate in Science and Education at the University of Pittsburgh. And, Zelda D. Johnson was the first to earn the Doctor of Pharmacy degree.

## *NIH/MBRS THEMATIC GRANT*

The thematic grant entitled "Chronopharmacological and Chronotherapeutic Investigations" funded in 1985, was instrumental in increasing the involvement of the College in chronopharmacological research and helped in establishing national and international recognition of the leading role of the FAMU College of Pharmacy in this research area. This grant (Table 8) also provided the opportunity for training of undergraduate and graduate students, as well as research fellows in chronopharmacology and chronotherapeutics.

Table 5. MBRS Principal Investigator, Funding Level, and Research Topics, 1973-1978.

| Principal Investigator | Research Topic | 1973-78 |
|---|---|---|
| Cottrel, P. T.[a] | Physical Chem. | $ 60,252 |
| Day, J. L. | Pharmaceutics | 118,688 |
| Lamba, S. S. | Synthetic/Natural Prod. Chem. | 57,042 |
| Ollapally, A. P.[a] | Synth. Organic Chem./Anti-Cancer | 164,327 |
| Shetty, A. S[b] | Biochemistry | 109,551 |
| Soliman, K. F. | Pharmacology | 92,612 |
| Trottier, R. W. | Pharmacology | 52,850 |
| Tterlikkis, L. P. | Pharmaceutics | 182,241 |
| Tterlikkis, L. P. | Administration Grant | 98,399 |
| | Total Direct Cost | $ 935,961 |
| | Indirect Cost | 32,975 |
| | Overall Total | $ 968,936 |

[a]Chemistry department.

[b]Biology department.

## *IMPACT OF THE MBRS PROGRAM ON THE DEVELOPMENT OF THE GRADUATE PROGRAM*

In the fall of 1971, Drs. Geraldine P. Woods and Charles A. Miller visited from the National Institutes of Health (NIH), Division of Basic Medical Sciences. Their mission was to explore the possibility of initiating a research program in predominantly black schools. In January 1972, Dr. Robert Gibbs from the NIH, Division of Research Resources visited and requested FAMU to submit a Comprehensive Institutional Research Proposal. The research proposal was submitted in February 1972 and research funds were awarded for five years beginning in the fall of 1973.

Discussion concerning a graduate program in science and engineering

Table 6. Tabulation of MBRS Students by Year.

| Year | Number of Graduate Students | Number of Undergraduate Students |
|---|---|---|
| 1973-83 | 4 | 153 |
| 1983-85 | 4 | 144 |
| 1985-87 | 5 | 97 |
| 1987-89 | 8 | 35 |
| 1989-91 | 12 | 36 |
| 1973-91 | 33 | 465 |
| Totals | 66 | 930 |

Table 7. Current Graduate and Undergraduate MBRS Students' Support.

| | Graduate | | Undergraduate |
|---|---|---|---|
| | MS | PhD | |
| Salary/Year | $7,500 | $8,500 | $6,000 |
| Tuition & Fees/Year | 2,300 | 2,300 | |
| Travel | 600 | 600 | 600 |
| Totals | $10,400 | $11,400 | $6,600 |

began in the spring of 1972, when the Office of Equal Opportunity visited with university faculty and administrators to assess future graduate programs at FAMU. In the same period, present Governor Lawton Chiles, then a U.S. Senator, visited the campus and met with faculty and administrators. The focus of his meeting was to support FAMU in securing a graduate program in the near future. Governor Chiles stated that "to have a viable graduate program, it is absolutely essential for the institution to have a strong research program."

In the fall of 1973, the School of Pharmacy's (the name was changed to College of Pharmacy and Pharmaceutical Sciences in 1983) administration and faculty were in a position to initiate a graduate program at the master of science level in pharmaceutical sciences. In the fall of 1975, a proposal was submitted to the Florida Board of Regents (BOR)

Table 8. NIH/MBRS Thematic Principal Investigators, Funding Level and Research Topics, 1985-1991.

| Principal Investigator | Research Topic | 1985-91 |
|---|---|---|
| Walker, C. A. | Administration | $ 13,560 |
| Walker, C. A. & Soliman, M. I. | Chronobiotic Drugs | 84,924 |
| Soliman, M. I. | Administration | 154,996 |
| Soliman, M. I. | Chronobiotic Drugs | 149,751 |
| Lee, H. J. | Chronopharmacology of Antiinflammatory steroids | 321,353 |
| | Total Direct Cost | $ 724,584 |
| | Indirect Cost | 248,540 |
| | Overall Total | $ 973,124 |

and subsequently approved for the masters program. In the summer of 1976, a graduate program in pharmacology/toxicology was initiated.

The effort to obtain Doctor of Philosophy (Ph.D.) programs at FAMU began with informal conversations between Dr. Charles Walker, Dean of the College of Pharmacy and Pharmaceutical Sciences and Dr. Charles U. Smith, Director of Graduate Studies. These two persons agreed in 1979-80 that in order for FAMU to achieve full peer status in the State University System and the appropriate recognition and level of respect in the national higher education community, advanced graduate degree programs were essential.

While four new master degree programs were added to FAMU's existing postgraduate programs in education during the middle and late 1970s, the institution was widely regarded, intramurally and extramurally, as basically an undergraduate school. Further, Walker and Smith were highly cognizant of the fact that FAMU was historically black and located just a few blocks from the predominantly white Florida State University (FSU), that already had many doctoral programs, that the BOR would not allow FAMU to duplicate.

Despite these obstacles, and knowing that the U.S. Office of Civil Rights had mandated that FAMU be allowed to establish curricula, programs, and degrees that would make it equal in attractiveness to FSU and the University of Florida, Drs. Walker and Smith proceeded to take their argument for Ph.D. programs to the FAMU Graduate Council. Resistance by some members of the Graduate Council, reflecting the traditional view of FAMU's scope and role, as well as a sense of futility about the BOR reaction, were soon abated, and turned into support for the Ph.D. initiatives when President Walter Smith gave his unqualified endorsement to the proposals.

In 1982, President Walter Smith was given approval by the BOR to prepare the first phase of the Ph.D. proposals for pharmacy and applied social science. Dr. Charles Walker, college dean coordinated the preparation of Phase I for the pharmacy Ph.D., and Dr. Charles U. Smith, graduate director and a sociologist was instrumental in the preparation of the proposal for their interdisciplinary social sciences Ph.D.

Recognizing the dearth of African American Ph.D.s in the sciences in general, and pharmacy specifically, the dean of the College of Pharmacy met with the President to set the stage for waging the perceived hard battle to establish FAMU's first doctor of philosophy degree.

As perceived it was not easy. Resistance, based on institutional mission which indicated no degrees for FAMU beyond the masters level made it more difficult. However, the tenacity of President Smith, Vice Presidents Gertrude Simmons, Leedell W. Neyland and former Dean Charles Walker to lead the fight, the endurance of the faculty and staff led by administrators like Drs. Johnnie L. Early, II and Henry Lewis, III provided basic support. Outstanding teaching and research results by faculty like Drs. Henry J. Lee, Maurice S. Holder, Karam F. A. Soliman, Surrendar S. Lamba, Arcelia Johnson-Fannin, Doris M. Stewart, and Thomas J. Fitzgerald reinforced the efforts.

Outstanding performance by the students on the licensure board helped the University and the College of Pharmacy and Pharmaceutical Sciences leadership to present a perfect case for the new degree program.

Ironically, the setting for the presentation was perfect. It was on the Florida A&M University campus, in the shiny new auditorium in the Ware-Rhaney building for Allied Health and Nursing that President Smith, Drs. Walker and Charles U. Smith made the first presentations (June 15, 1983) and participated in the debate in support of the proposed new program with the BOR Program Committee, chaired by Regent William Malloy. Dr. Walker had the foresight to make quiet contact with the Academic Program office of the BOR, prior to the formal presentations. After discussion, Regent Malloy relinquished the chair, and made the motion to approve the 2 Ph.D. program requests, which was assessed by the Program Committee. In the afternoon, following the recommendation of the BOR Program Committee, the full BOR approved planning for Phase II of the 2 programs.

Cooperative planning did take place. Over the next year, plans, strategies, and ensuing battles to overcome the resistant Post Secondary Education Planning Commission (PEPC) were waged. The BOR was a participant early on and remained steadfast throughout. Dr. Tribble, the Associate Vice Chancellor for Academic Programs was the key contact person for the BOR.

FAMU students performed outstandingly at the National MBRS Symposium in Washington, DC, in part, as an outcome of their participation in the Student Research Forum. The Student Research Forum was initiated by the Assistant Dean for Research and MBRS Program Director in 1981. And, the Forum under the leadership of the current MBRS Program Director, continues to prepare students for national meetings. FAMU graduates maintained high passing marks on the boards, and Dr. Henry Lee announced that his "steroids" research was ready for patent application and publication.

These activities coupled with a high visibility reception at the president's residence for Dr. Hans Mark, Deputy Administrator of NASA where Dr. Mark announced FAMU's special role in NASA's motion sickness research program, a $300,000 commitment by Warner-Lambert Pharmaceutical Company to help fund an Eminent Scholar's Chair in the Pharmaceutical Sciences, increased NIH funding, and the receipt of an endowment funded by the Plough Foundation for professional student scholarships, made the final battles easier.

Dr. Charles A. Walker, former Chancellor of the University of Arkansas at Pine Bluff, was very instrumental in the initiation of the Ph.D. program in 1985 and reflected on the struggle:

> It was very difficult because there were people who felt at that time, that a doctoral program of any kind should probably not be at FAMU. But now, we're finding that with the tremendous decrease of minorities earning the Ph.D. in the basic sciences, that the Ph.D. programs at predominately African American institutions are very significant and are going to become even more significant in the future as the need for Ph.D. level scientists is going to be required in the workforce.

In January 1984, the BOR authorized FAMU to plan a new Ph.D. program in pharmaceutical sciences with specialization in pharmacology/toxicology. Two independent consultants were contracted by the BOR to review the College's request for authorization to conduct a feasibility study, and to conduct site visits. The evaluations of the consultants, Dr. Hugh F. Kabat, College of Pharmacy, University of Minnesota, now with the University of New Mexico, College of Pharmacy, Albuquerque, NM and Dr. John W. Schermerhorn, Dean, College of Allied Health Sciences, University of Texas, Health Sciences Center, Dallas, TX, supported the development of the proposed program with no qualifications or reservations. The BOR staff recommended that authorization be given to plan the program.

On July 13, 1984, the 13 member BOR, with Dr. Barbara Newell, Chancellor, and Attorney Robin Gibson, Chairman, approved the Ph.D. program for implementation in January 1985 with any additional resources to be obtained through reallocation of existing sources. Four tracks were approved: pharmacology/toxicology, medicinal chemistry, pharmaceutics, and pharmacy administration. In giving its approval, the Board of Regents noted that the M.S. program had been designated by the Regents as a Program of Emphasis; graduate research capabilities of the College are commensurate with Ph.D. level training; and the realization that more than 50% of the M.S. graduates were continuing their education in Ph.D. and M.D. programs elsewhere.

Changes in the composition of BOR, with new perspectives among its membership resulted in a reversal of the final planning and implementation of the Ph.D. in applied social sciences.

After BOR approval, the next step required concurrence from the PEPC. PEPC listened to the presentations and struggled with the evidence and the weight of the BOR decision. PEPC decided that the BOR decision was inconsistent with the overall statewide plan. The vote was a divided no on the Ph.D. program. The issue was referred back to the BOR at their next meeting and it then received a unanimous vote and implementation began.

## *DEVELOPMENT OF THE PH.D. TRACK IN ENVIRONMENTAL TOXICOLOGY*

A Cooperative Agreement was implemented between the Centers for Disease Control, Agency for Toxic Substances and Disease Registry (ATSDR), and the eight member Association of Minority Health Professions Schools in 1988. The agreement focuses on the health problems of minorities through the application of the considerable research and training capabilities of minority health professions schools. The agreement currently encompasses: research in toxicology, risk assessment, and a Ph.D. program in environmental toxicology at FAMU.

The College received funding to form an advisory committee, composed of toxicologists from ATSDR, academia, Battelle Laboratories, Seattle, Washington, the National Center for Toxicological Research, and FAMU. The resulting curriculum was established in August 1990, and both the recruitment and enrollment of students proceeded. Funding for a fellowship was secured through a competitive grant from the U.S. Department of Energy.

The national impact of the graduate program was illustrated with the April 1991 graduation of five African Americans with the Ph.D. in the pharmaceutical sciences. This was the first occurrence, among the 61 pharmacy schools with graduate programs, of such a number of African Americans simultaneously graduating. FAMU has graduated seven Ph.D.s through 1991 (Figure 1). According to the American Association of College of Pharmacy statistics, only 14 African Americans received their Ph.D. degree from 1984 through 1989, or an annual average of 2.8. The future admissions to the program appear positive as the number of applications since the implementation of the Ph.D. program have increased (Figure 2).

The intensive recruitment efforts for graduate students have been further augmented by the assistance of both the Florida Endowment Fund and Upjohn. Prospective students and their mentors are invited to attend a Colloquium on Graduate Pharmaceutical education during the MBRS/Minority Access to Research Careers Symposium, and the National Institute of Science, Beta Kappa Chi Convention. The students are given a graduate program and Florida Endowment Fund program overview, and a scientific presentation by a current McKnight Fellow. Faculty and graduate students then discuss the program with prospective students. A key feature of the graduate program is the requirement for both presentations and publications. At the masters level, students are required to submit a paper for publication in a refereed journal, and to present a paper at a national scientific meeting. At the Ph.D. level, two publications and presentations are required. The rate of publications with graduate student authors or coauthors (Figure 3) has grown steadily from two in 1983 to ten in 1989 and nine in 1990. Presentations numbered 20 in 1984, 16 in 1989, and 27 in 1990.

The research of each graduate student was supported by both the MBRS and RCMI programs. A NASA grant partially supported two (Hyacinth Akunne and Ebenezer Oriaku) students. All were MBRS trainees at the beginning of their studies, but three (Marcus B. Iszard, Joyce V. Lee, and

Figure 1. NUMBER OF GRADUATE DEGREES AWARDED

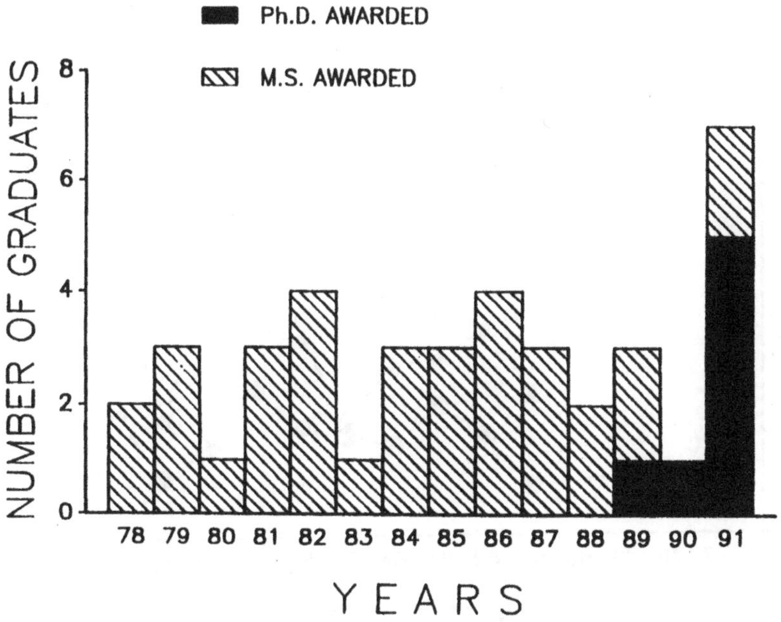


Robert Williams) graduated as McKnight Fellows (see the Florida Endowment Fund for Higher Education, below). One (Hugh M. McLean), was supported by a Patricia Roberts-Harris Fellowship (see the Patricia Roberts-Harris Fellowship Program, below) and a 3M Scholarship. The seven graduates have entered postdoctoral training (National Institute of Mental Health, National Center for Toxicological Research, Pfizer Pharmaceuticals, University of Kansas Medical Center), assumed positions in the pharmaceutical industry (3M Pharmaceuticals, Parke-Davis), in academia (FAMU and the University of Arkansas at Pine Bluff) and the federal government (Agency for Toxic Substances and Disease Registry).

## *FELLOWSHIPS*

The College has benefitted tremendously from several federal, state, foundation, and corporate mechanisms of graduate and Pharm.D. student support. Each mechanism brings prestige to both the recipient and the College. And, more importantly, stability to the graduate program which

Figure 2. GRADUATE STUDENT APPLICATIONS

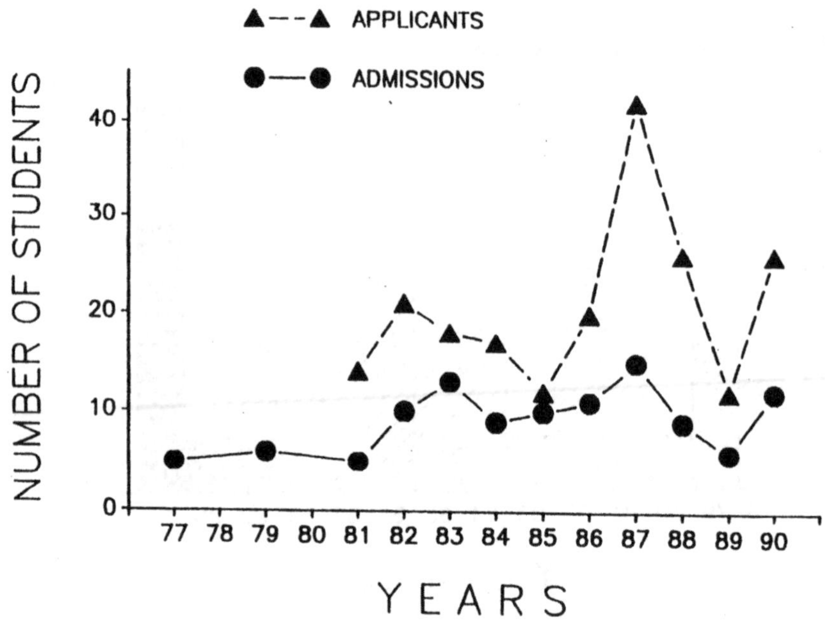


is highly dependent on extramural sources of support. The retention of graduate students is undoubtedly enhanced by this support.

## THE FLORIDA ENDOWMENT FUND FOR HIGHER EDUCATION

The Florida Endowment Fund (FEF) for Higher Education was established as a result of a dialogue and synergy between political leadership and all sectors of higher education in the State of Florida. An agreement was reached in 1983 that led to the development of an agenda for the advancement of higher education which would project Florida well into the 21st Century.

One of the main features of FEF is the McKnight Doctoral Fellowship Program which supports African-American students pursuing the Ph.D. degree. The program provides initially up to 69 fellows to pursue Ph.D.s in the State of Florida.

Figure 3. GRADUATE STUDENT PRESENTATIONS AND PUBLICATIONS

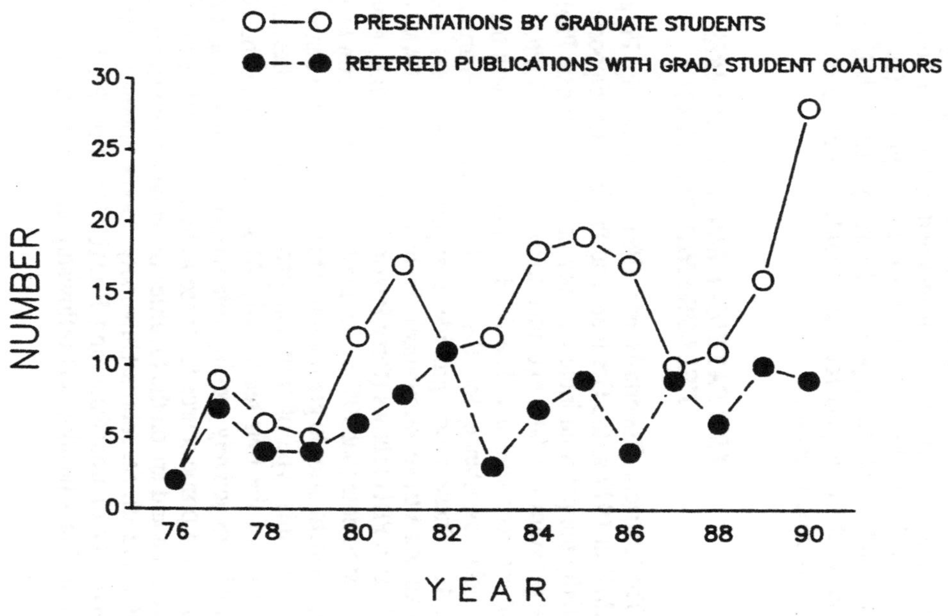

Florida A&M University has received support for twelve African-American Ph.D. candidates (6 males and 6 females) between the years of 1985-91. The FEF program has lost only one student of the twelve who have been supported to give a retention rate of 92 percent. Statewide, McKnight Fellows have been retained at a rate of 86 percent. The FEF provides $15,000/year support for each student (stipend, tuition fees, books and travel) for a period of three years. FAMU then provides the same level of support for the candidate until he or she completes the Ph.D. degree program.

## *THE PATRICIA ROBERTS-HARRIS FELLOWSHIP PROGRAM*

The Patricia Roberts-Harris (PRH) Fellowship Program began at FAMU in 1979 as the Graduate and Professional Opportunities Program. Initially the program included only postbaccalaureate Pharm.D. students. The program was later extended to include the M.S./Ph.D. in pharmaceutical sciences students. The PRH funding is and was the only source of financial assistance for the Postbaccalaureate Pharm.D. students at FAMU. These funds provide a stipend of $10,000 annually (tuition, books and a travel allowance). To date 1979-1991, FAMU has graduated forty-two PRH fellows (forty Pharm.D. and two Ph.D. graduates). It is of interest to note that 90% of the graduates of the Pharm.D. program found employment prior to graduation. This speaks for the demand for individuals with this type of training, particularly minorities. In addition, the faculties of the four historically African American and other pharmacy schools are actively seeking role models for their programs, and FAMU has been a prime source for these individuals. PRH Fellows from FAMU have been and are on the faculties of: Howard University, The University of Cincinnati, St. John's University, Texas Southern University, Xavier University of Louisiana, and FAMU. The first PRH Ph.D. graduate is completing a postdoctoral fellowship at Pfizer Pharmaceuticals.

## *AMERICAN FOUNDATION FOR PHARMACEUTICAL EDUCATION FELLOWSHIP AND DELORES AUZENNE SCHOLARSHIP*

Important graduate student support is also received from the American Foundation for Pharmaceutical Education (AFPE). A Ph.D. student has received a regular fellowship of $6,000 in 1990, and a Sydnor Barksdale

Penick Memorial Fellowship of $4,000 in 1991. Others have received the Delores Auzenne Scholarship ($5,000), a State of Florida program for minority graduate students.

## *RESEARCH CENTERS AT MINORITY INSTITUTIONS: PROVISION OF ESSENTIAL INFRASTRUCTURE SUPPORT*

The Research Centers at Minority Institutions Program was established on July 26, 1984 by the Labor, Health and Human Services, and Education and Related Agencies Appropriation Bill (H.R. 6028). The House Report (pages 78, 79) on the FY 1985 referenced the Secretary's most recent annual report on Health in the U.S., which focused renewed attention on disparities in health status between minority and white Americans. The RCMI Program is designed to expand the national capability for research in the health sciences by assisting, through grant support, predominantly minority institutions that offer the doctorate in the health professions and/or health-related sciences. The RCMI Program is intended to enhance significantly the capacity for the conduct of biomedical and/or behavioral research at such minority institutions by strengthening their research environment. To be eligible to participate, an institution must have more than 50 percent minority student enrollment, award an M.D., a DDS, a D.V.M. or other doctoral degree in the health professions and/or a Ph.D. in the sciences related to health. FAMU offers both the Doctor of Pharmacy and Ph.D. degrees.

### *Support Staff*

A key component of the FAMU RCMI program is the provision of staff which are essential to the research infrastructure. In addition to well-trained and experienced research support office staff, there is a statistician who reviews the experimental design, and assists with the evaluation of data. His skill eliminates the common errors of: excessive numbers of animals, poor design and inappropriate statistical tests. The scientific editor's skill has increased clarity and completeness, reduced the criticism of grammatical errors, and along with word processing programs, the presence of numerous typographical errors which detract from the readability and competitiveness of proposals. The art editor has significantly improved our capability in producing high quality graphics for both publications and presentations. While some needs are met through computer programs, many require the human touch. In each instance, the presence of such personnel not only improves the quality of proposals and the like, but they also reduce the time and cost of production in contrast to wherewithal required by ad hoc consultants.

### *Research Associates*

The primary goal of this RCMI activity is to provide research experiences for minority recipients of the Ph.D., D.V.M., M.D. and Pharm.D. degrees in pharmacology/toxicology, pharmaceutics, and clinical pharmacy. Both the research capability of the College and the competitiveness of the involved faculty member should be enhanced. Moreover, the nation should benefit from the emergence of both basic and clinical scientists who have strengthened their research capability through an intensive research experience.

The selection of the faculty to whom a research associate is to be assigned is determined by a peer committee based on the following criteria. The investigator should: (1) have a viable research program as evidenced by: (a) funded research grant(s); (b) refereed publications from research completed at FAMU in the last two years; and (c) published abstracts or presentations during the last two years; (2) the absence of research associate position on any other grant; and (3) engagement in research activity which is expected to lead to a proposal. Research associate appointments are two years in duration.

The selection of the research associate is based on the following criteria: (1) the applicant must have a doctoral degree (Ph.D., Pharm.D., M.D. or D.V.M.); (2) the time between the research associate's graduation date and FAMU's appointment should not exceed three years; and (3) the applicant should be recommended by three persons with whom he/she has had contact. A research associate is expected to: perform research work which is of high caliber; publish or present research work at national meetings; and generate data which can be utilized in writing research proposals.

### *Impact of Research Associates on the Faculty*

Faculty who obtained research associates increased their publication rate in the period 1985-1990. When comparing the faculty members that have research associates working in their labs with those who do not, six faculty members who had RCMI supported research associates published

44 papers during the last two years, an average of 7.33 publications per faculty member. The eighteen faculty members without RCMI supported research associates published only eleven papers. This gave them an average of 0.61 papers per faculty.

### *Impact of Research Associates on the National Need for Biomedical Scientists*

Two research associates are now faculty members at minority institutions. One is currently assistant professor of pharmaceutics at the College of Pharmacy and Pharmaceutical Sciences, Howard University, and the other is currently an associate professor of toxicology at the University of Arkansas at Pine Bluff.

### *Research Productivity*

During the period from 1983 to 1987, there was an average of about nineteen published, refereed papers annually by pharmacy faculty (Figure 4). Since initiation of the RCMI grant in October, 1985, there has been a great increase in the research activity. In 1988, there were twenty-one publications, an increase of about 11 percent more than the previous five-year average. This increase in publications for 1988 reflects the beginning of published data generated by the RCMI grant.

In 1990, faculty published 26 refereed articles. In 1989, there were 36 publications, an increase of about 89 percent over the 1983 to 1987 yearly average. During 1988-1989, when the influence of the RCMI grant on the publications rate could first be seen, the faculty published 57 papers. Since there are 24 faculty members, there was an average of 2.4 publications per faculty member. The six faculty members who had RCMI supported faculty development experience opportunities, published 15 papers with an overall average of 2.5 publications per faculty member during the last two years. Thus, the RCMI grant has significantly boosted the rate of publications in the College.

### *Grant Applications Submitted*

The number of research grants awarded increased from five grants in 1983 to 30 awarded in 1990 (Figure 5). This increase reflects the impact

Figure 4. FACULTY PUBLICATIONS

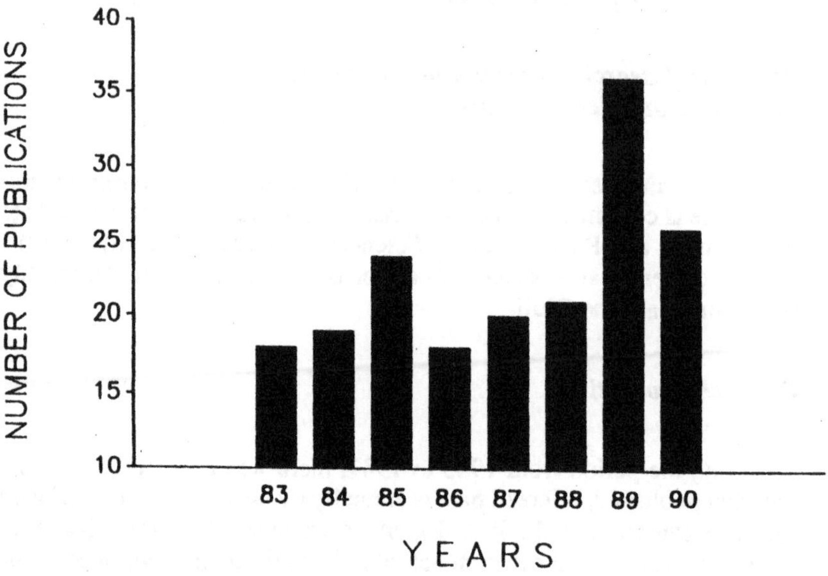


of the presubmission review procedure that started in 1981, and the Ph.D. program which was approved in 1984, but started in 1985. The actual grant support increased from $600,000 in 1983 to $3.7 million in 1990 (Figure 6).

### *Library Resources*

The College of Pharmacy Library is a branch library of the Samuel H. Coleman Library at Florida Agricultural and Mechanical University. It is physically located within the College of Pharmacy in the Clifton G. Dyson Building, room 200. Until 1985, nearly all of the costs of the program were absorbed by the Coleman Library. With the advent of RCMI funding in 1985, several major alterations took place in the College of Pharmacy Library environment.

The RCMI funds impacted significantly on the quality of services available to students during extended hours. Until RCMI, library staff

Figure 5. GRANTS AWARDED

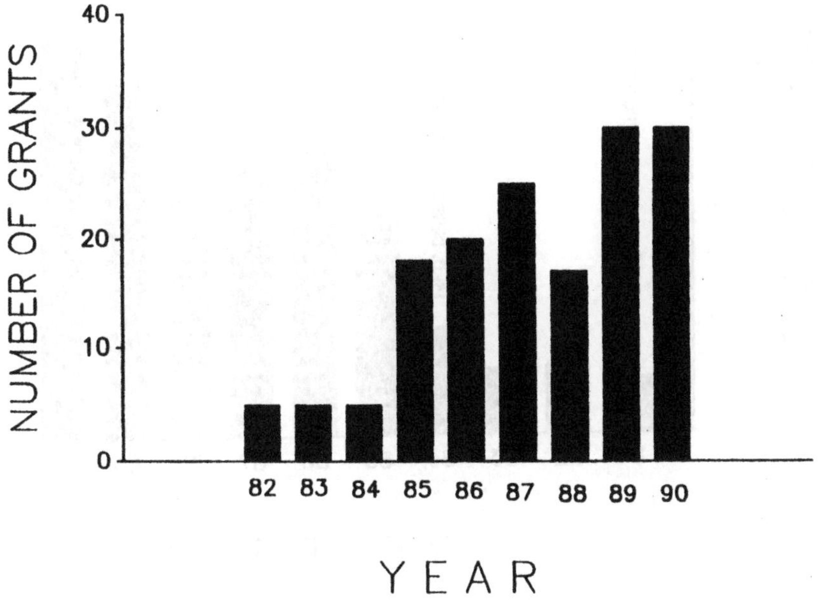


was limited to one professional librarian assigned by the Coleman Library. Extended hours beyond the 40 hours provided for by Coleman Library were operated using graduate pharmacy school students. Coleman Library also provided funds for several FAMU student assistants to help the librarian with routine tasks. RCMI funds were used to employ two, part-time professional librarians and one clerical assistant during nights and weekend open hours. Students now have access to the full range of professional librarian research assistance during all library open hours of operation.

Projects to provide on-line computerized searching and free end-user database searching were initiated and developed using the RCMI funds. The library now offers on-line searching of medical and health sciences literature to FAMU students and faculty. Subscriptions to DIALOG online databases, MEDLINE on CDROM, DRUGDEX, and POISINDEX Computerized Clinical Information System (CCIS) on CDROM are cur-

Figure 6. GRANT SUPPORT

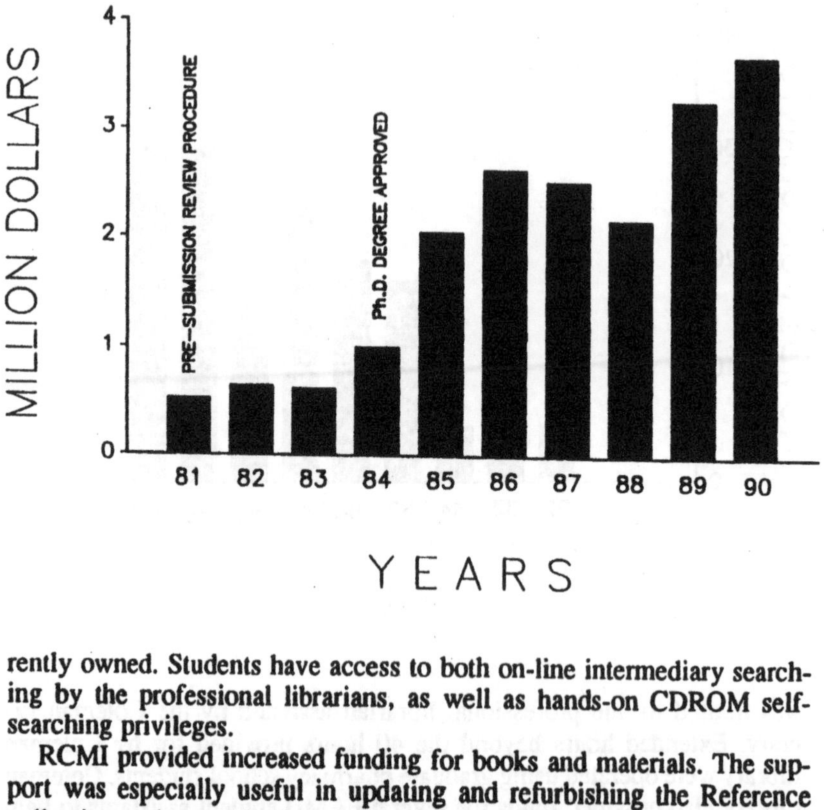


rently owned. Students have access to both on-line intermediary searching by the professional librarians, as well as hands-on CDROM self-searching privileges.

RCMI provided increased funding for books and materials. The support was especially useful in updating and refurbishing the Reference collection and strengthening pharmacology and toxicology library books holdings on the graduate level. Expensive reference texts held at Coleman Library are seldom duplicated in branch libraries, especially titles that are multidisciplinary in subject treatment. As a result of the policy, general encyclopedias and dictionaries as well as multidisciplinary health science materials basic to reference and research needs were out-of-date or nonexistent in the Pharmacy Library. RCMI funds were used to purchase these as well as duplicate volumes of heavily used reserve books.

Phase I of a project to replace missing issues of journals held was realized. The funds provided for purchase of journals on microfilm reels covering issues missing from volumes for titles A through J. The library currently has full runs of back issues for more than half of the titles that were recorded on the missing issues list.

The following is a breakdown of biomedical books added since 1978.

| Year | Number of Books Added |
|---|---|
| 1979-80 | 927 |
| 1980-81 | 125 |
| 1981-82 | 18 |
| 1982-83 | 563 |
| 1983-84 | 783 |
| 1984-85 | 847 |
| 1985-86 | 567 |
| 1986-87 | 281 |
| 1987-88 | 802 |
| 1988-89 | 614 |
| 1989-90 | 419 |
| Total | 5,946 |

This total increases the current monograph holdings to 14,487 biomedical books. Approximately ten percent of the annual increases in monograph volumes are attributable to RCMI expenditures.

### *Laboratory Animal Facility*

The laboratory animal facility in the Dyson Pharmacy Building was renovated and upgraded to meet all PHS and NIH guidelines. An additional two rooms were added to this facility for housing animals used in chronopharmacological research. A satellite animal suite was also renovated in the Psychology Department of the Gore Education Building. The animal holding area increased in Dyson Pharmacy Building from 570 to 1,111 square feet and the ventilation system upgraded to 15 air changes per hour. The facility is also supported by an emergency generator. These renovations, upgrading and additions were made possible through funds provided by RCMI, MBRS, and institutional funds. Through the MBRS supplemental grant (#RR08111) of $100,000, new areas were added including a storage room and the ventilation system was upgraded to provide the required air exchanges. In addition, MBRS funds were allocated to provide one-month training of the animal facility supervisor at the University of Florida animal facility which is AAALAC accredited. This training was beneficial in improving the operational procedures of the facility to provide excellent animal husbandry. Additional cages and racks were purchased through RCMI funds.

In order to increase the efficient utilization of space for housing animals, Duo-Flo units and ventilated racks are being purchased through funds provided by RCMI grant. These expansions resulted in doubling the animal holding capability and helped in meeting the increasing laboratory animal needs for research. There are currently three operational animal facilities on campus. Two facilities are located in Dyson Pharmacy Building (DPB). The DPB facilities include two rooms designed to house animals used in chronopharmocological research. The third facility (420 sq. ft.) is located in the Psychology Department. All three facilities conform with PHS guidelines and regulations and are controlled for lighting, humidity and temperature. The HVAC system of DPB facilities is supported by a functioning emergency generator.

### *Chemical Storeroom*

The RCMI program funded the establishment of the first chemical storeroom on campus. This is a centralized facility used for the procurement of over 200 chemicals, a wide selection of glassware, and a limited offering of surgical supplies. Investigators can now avoid the time delay previously associated with procurement of common supply items. The storeroom also facilitates the service ordering directly, via computer modem, from vendors (Sigma and Fisher).

### *Instrumentation Grant*

Through an instrumentation grant from NIH/MBRS, it was possible to purchase a state-of-the-art LKB liquid scintillation counter. This instrument is extensively used by many investigators and their graduate students working with radioisotopes in metabolism studies and receptor assays. Moreover, both the MBRS and RCMI programs have provided equipment necessary for the conduct of research. While the MBRS program primarily provided equipment for specific research projects, RCMI provided major equipment which is essential for a competitive research environment. Among the major items of equipment are 60mHz NMR and an IR to enable researchers to identify new compounds. An explosion proof fume hood was installed, and existing fume hoods were repaired and/or adjusted. The College is now equipped with centrifuges, spectrophotometers and HPLCs to meet the basic research needs of the community.

Audiovisual equipment was acquired to allow the art editor to prepare high quality charts, graphs and photographs. A donation from 3M provided for some equipment. The College renovated space to accommodate this service. Both the Upjohn Company and the Merck Company Foundation have provided support for equipment.

### *Clinical Pharmacology Research Unit*

The Clinical Pharmacology Research Unit (CPRU), located in Miami, Florida, is a core laboratory open to all FAMU faculty members and students, and to other collaborators. It is supported by both FAMU and the RCMI grant for the purpose of conducting human drug studies. Staffing includes an M.D./Ph.D., administrative assistant, nurse, and an analytical chemist.

The future of graduate pharmaceutical education and research appears bright at FAMU because of three factors. President Humphries not only urges students to enter graduate and professional schools, he has implemented a graduate feeder program with 25 universities. The feeder program serves as a key and effective means of interfacing on behalf of students, with graduate and professional degree providers. This program will further promote the tradition of graduate study among our students (2). A key development is the acceptance of a 1991 B.S. pharmacy graduate for admission in the fall semester, 1991, and, the announcements of other pharmacy students of their intent to apply beginning in 1991. Both President Humphries and Provost and Vice President Richard A. Hogg, scientists in their own right, are aggressively supporting both research, and the development of graduate programs in the sciences. The provision of state lines and fiscal resources promote greater achievements. Moreover, key decisions by President Humphries, who is also the RCMI principal investigator, have created an enhanced research environment.

Second, the construction of the basic science research building is planned in 1992 for a $10.9 million 59,210 sq. ft. facility. The College will occupy 11,440 sq. ft. (if the legislature provides funding as requested). At this writing, we are assured of only $6 million. Clearly, the success of the College played a key role in the approval of this facility, the first in this decade, and the first new building on the FAMU campus since 1985.

Third, the success of the College attracted yet another major contribution to its effort. On February 16, 1989, the University's first endowed chair was established in the College through the contributions of the Warner Lambert Company ($300,000), FAMU's Centennial Campaign

($300,000), and the State of Florida ($400,000). The Warner Lambert Eminent Scholar Chair in the Biomedical Sciences will be utilized to further develop an academic and research program of international distinction.

## *CONCLUSIONS*

Since the first MBRS award, extramural federal support has been essential to the development and growth of both research and graduate pharmaceutical research at FAMU. Support of fellowships and scholarships by foundations, federal programs, and pharmaceutical manufacturers fills the gap between state funding and needs. Graduate pharmaceutical education exists because of a receptive Board of Regents, a capable faculty, visionary and determined college talented students, administrators, supportive central administration, *and* extramural support. These factors have enabled the College to become the nation's preeminent provider of African Americans with the Ph.D. degree in the pharmaceutical sciences.

Similarly, the College has become more competitive in securing extramural funds due to the maturation afforded by the MBRS program and the infrastructure provided by the RCMI program. The MBRS program formed the essential foundation for research and graduate pharmaceutical education. Clearly, the College was well prepared in 1984 to implement a Ph.D. program, on the strength of an MBRS award which included twelve subprojects versus six in the 1980 grant, and was funded at $535,000 or a 250 percent increase over the previous award. The RCMI program has enabled the College beyond the resources provided by state appropriations. Moreover, in comparing the College with other pharmacy schools, which receive NIH biomedical research support grant awards, the College now ranks number eleven with $1.7 million in NIH funding.

It is evident from the data presented, beginning in 1973, that African American institutions can achieve in the research arena when provided with the opportunity and support. It is also evident that HBCUs play a vital role in the correction of the underrepresentation of minorities at the Ph.D. level in the biomedical sciences.

## ACKNOWLEDGMENTS

Special thanks and acknowledgement are given to Glory B. Brown, Program Assistant; DeNise Gordon, Art Editor; Frances James, Grants

Coordinator; and O. Sylvia Lamar, Scientific Editor. This document was supported by grants (NIH/NCRR/RCMI #GM03020, NIH/NIGMS/MBRS #GM08111, RAP/NCRR, NIH #RR03196, NASA #NAG411, NASA/Cosmos #K6-19 and K7-19, and NIH/NIGMS/MBRS Thematic #GM02660). The support of the graduate program by the American Foundation for Pharmaceutical Education, ATSDR, The Upjohn Company, Pfizer Central Research, 3M Foundation, The Merck Company Foundation, The Florida Endowment Fund, Patricia Roberts-Harris, Delores Auzenne Scholarship Program, Warner-Lambert, Department of Energy Fellowship Program #DE-FG05-89ER 75523, and The Procter & Gamble Company Research and Development Department, is gratefully acknowledged. The support of the National Science Foundation #IRS 59-0977035 is also gratefully acknowledged.

## REFERENCES

1. Early JL, Walker CA. Increasing research proposal funding competitiveness. In: Okolo EN, ed. Health research design and methodology. Boca Raton, FL: CRC Press, 1990:15-9.

2. Brazziel WF. Baccalaureate college of origin of Black doctorate recipients. J Negro Educ 1983;52:102-9.

# Barriers to a Career in Pharmacy: An Hispanic Perspective

Carmen Aceves-Blumenthal

**SUMMARY.** The underrepresentation of minority and Hispanic students in the pharmacy profession not only reflects the inequities in access to this profession, but also a maldistribution of pharmacy services to the minority population. Financial, cultural and motivational issues play a part in impeding the accession of more Hispanic students into the profession of pharmacy. A lack of role models and professional images of pharmacy also act as barriers to the selection of pharmacy as a career option. Real or self-imposed language barriers restrict a student's performance in the standardized PCAT examination as well as in didactic and clinical course work. The APhA proposes vigorous, long-term programs in recruitment, establishing a network of minority role models and the development of recruitment guidelines for colleges of pharmacy.

The purpose of this article is to provide an overview of some of the issues impacting on minority and, specifically, Hispanic student entry into the pharmacy profession. There is a paucity of information addressing this issue. Studies that have looked at minority student characteristics, motivation for seeking careers in pharmacy and recruitment tools for minority students can be counted on one hand. All authors admit that there are low numbers of minority pharmacists and/or students in pharmacy (1-3).

The issue of underrepresentation of minorities in the health professions

Carmen Aceves-Blumenthal, B.S.Pharm., M.S., is Director of Experiential Education and Assistant Professor of Pharmacy Practice at the Southeastern University of the Health Sciences College of Pharmacy, 1750 N.E. 168th Street, North Miami Beach, FL 33181. She is also Adjunct Assistant Professor of Family Medicine at the Southeastern University of the Health Sciences College of Osteopathic Medicine.

 

has come of age. It has been identified as one of the priorities to be addressed by the 1991 American Pharmaceutical Association (APhA), House of Delegates at its annual meeting in New Orleans.

Equity in education is not the only reason for the increased awareness for the need to increase minority participation in the health professions. Equity in access to health care by the minority population of our society is another reason for concern. Walker suggests that the low number of minority pharmacists results in a maldistribution of pharmacy services to minorities in our society. His figures indicate that in 1972, only 2,400 of the 121,000 (1.98%) of the licensed pharmacists in the United States were Black (2). This observation is reinforced by Weinert et al., who conclude that minority pharmacy graduates are more likely to pursue careers in minority environments than their nonminority counterparts (4).

Hispanic membership in the profession of pharmacy has also been well below what one might expect from such a prominent sector of our population. A review of the number of degrees conferred on Hispanic students from 1976 through 1988 reveals that a total of 111,057 Baccalaureate and Doctoral pharmacy degrees were awarded. Only 4,388 or 3.95% of all degrees were awarded to Hispanic students (5).

The Educational Affairs Policy Committee for the APhA has cited several reasons for the scarcity of minority students in the profession. Among the reasons identified were:

- high cost of education
- lack of scholarship programs
- image that pharmacy is not an active participant in health care
- lack of minority role models in pharmacy
- lack of awareness of pharmacy as a profession (1).

These reasons have been echoed by other authors addressing the issue of minority education in the health professions. For minorities in our society, the realities of daily life and scarcity of resources sometimes serve as absolute barriers and limit the length, extent and possibilities of higher education (6). The choice between utilization of family resources for survival versus the "luxury" of investing in the future (in the form of professional education) is brutally clear. The financial burden of formal pharmacy education often limits this profession to the wealthy few. However, there are other factors that influence the selection of a career in pharmacy.

The image of pharmacy within the Hispanic community, according to the Educational Affairs Policy Committee, is "as a drug-keeper, a businessman whose drugs are overpriced . . . usually not an active participant in a community's health care" (1). Such unfavorable views of pharmacy would certainly preclude it as a choice for members of that culture.

A study of Mexican-American pharmacy students by Hanson and Kirk also emphasizes the cultural impact on the perception of pharmacists. Their study indicates that Hispanics may hesitate in seeking health care due to cultural dissimilarities between Hispanics and health care providers (3). Avoiding interactions with health professionals, or seeing only Anglos in those roles does not reinforce these professions as viable alternatives to the Hispanic student.

Career alternatives, even for those few Hispanics that manage to enter the profession of pharmacy, are also limited. Hanson and Kirk pointed out that the primary goal of Mexican-American pharmacy students was to own a community pharmacy. They indicated that this goal was most prevalent because it is the role with which these students were most familiar (3).

There is relatively little information regarding the images that people in our society have on the various professions. The image problem that pharmacy has is not limited to the Hispanic culture. Poirier and Lipetz, in their description of a course on images of health professions in the media, emphasize the lack of images of pharmacists in the media (7). They relate that even when an issue was directly related to pharmacy, the media generally selected physicians, research scientists, or pharmaceutical company spokespeople as the drug experts (7).

In our materialistic and success-oriented society, image and prestige of occupations play a role in career selection. An occupation's prestige is generally ascribed by its image in society. One would predict that young people would select high prestige professions more often than not (8). However, occupational prestige in itself may serve as another barrier to health care professions education for minority students. Although higher education, and, specifically, health professions education, may promote a great deal of economic progress, high levels of social conflict can emerge due to the dichotomies between cultures (9). Potential students may feel that by selecting a high prestige occupation, they are stating their dissatisfaction with their cultural heritage and family life-style. Rather than turn their backs on their culture, they may select occupations that are more congruent with their social norms.

Further, for a person to select a career, the expected occupational role must be congruent with the person's concept of self (8). Therefore, selection of a career must be consistent with the self-picture. If Hispanics do not see themselves as pharmacists, they will not become pharmacists.

Anticipated failure or the perception that the minority student will not be successful in completing professional program requirements adds to the barriers in career selection (2).

In addition to barriers in selecting pharmacy as a career, there are barriers to minority and Hispanic students in the admissions process. Educators have become increasingly aware of the limitations in interpreting the results of standardized examinations. Critics claim that these examinations are culturally biased toward the middle-class white student. This bias may also be observed in performance levels in the Pharmacy College Admissions Test (PCAT). Based upon generalizations from other standardized examinations, it could be predicted that minority students will score lower in the reading and verbal abilities section of this exam. In fact, at Southeastern University of the Health Sciences, College of Pharmacy, where 31% of the applicants for academic year 1991/92 are Hispanic, verbal ability and reading scores are often well below the fiftieth percentile. However, upon interviewing the candidate, significant language deficiencies are not apparent. Hence, PCAT scores used in conjunction with other admission criteria can serve as another barrier to admission.

Once enrolled in a pharmacy curriculum, minority and Hispanic students are faced with other barriers. As already mentioned, the cultural perception of health care and the role of the pharmacist within the health care system will impact on an Hispanic student's perception of their future professional role. If they see the role of the pharmacist as limited to community practice, they will only aspire to that role. Walker's study showed that minority students (Black, Hispanic or American Indian), were generally unaware of career opportunities in pharmacy outside of the traditional community and hospital settings (2).

These role limitations can impact on the extent to which students perform in a variety of courses. If the student does not perceive benefit to the subject under study, the tendency is to ignore and not internalize that material, thus leading to mediocre academic performance.

One of the areas of importance in pharmacy education is training students for effective patient counseling. Counseling is the most important and most difficult skill for the health care professional to master. It involves the sharing of concerns regarding feelings and problems, and requires active listening by the participants (10). Effective communication requires that students learn to interact with others at various levels: whether with a patient, other student, college faculty or other health care professionals. Interactions and patient counseling can be either in written or oral format, but most often involve both types.

Some Hispanic students exhibit real or self-imposed language barriers.

For students where English is a second language, this barrier can be very real. The differences in terminology, the varying level of sophistication in both written and oral communication techniques as well as lack of understanding, dramatically impact on student performance, especially in the more clinical, patient-oriented courses.

Self-imposed language barriers are seen in students who are uncomfortable with their accent or are unsure of their vocabulary. Often, this self-imposed barrier impedes the student's progress. College-based faculty, as well as preceptors in experiential rotations, may misinterpret the student's hesitancy as a sign of being unprepared or lacking sufficient knowledge.

Further, students with language barriers have a tendency to assume a nonassertive communication style. This style implies a negative self-worth and is generally inappropriate when dealing with patients and other health care practitioners (10). Students need to communicate in an assertive manner; a manner where personal desires and goals are stated without infringing on others (10). This style, however, must be learned and practiced for the student to become comfortable with it.

The conversion of highly technical medical jargon into patient-oriented language is also a barrier observed in patient education. English speaking students have difficulty expressing technical concepts they have learned in school to the average lay patient. On the other hand, bilingual students may be most effective in the provision of health care and counseling patients of similar ethnic background. As with their English speaking counterparts, however, translation of technical medical terms learned in English into patient-oriented language poses the initial barrier. Compounding this barrier is the need to translate patient instructions into a different language.

Having identified some of the barriers to minority enrollment and success in pharmacy programs, how can we begin to address these issues?

Recommendations from the APhA Policy Committee on Educational Affairs include that the APhA:

1. support a vigorous long-term program for recruitment of minority students into the profession.
2. encourage the development and updating of comprehensive minority-aimed recruitment materials.
3. encourage professional association at the local, state and national level to create a network of minority pharmacist role models.
4. support the development of minority recruitment guidelines for colleges of pharmacy (1).

These recommendations, from a national pharmacy organization, are seen as steps in increasing national and professional awareness of these issues. The difficulty arises in the implementation of these recommendations. How do we get more minority students interested in pharmacy? How can we recruit them into our profession? Are scholarship monies available to help defray the cost of a pharmacy education? Will more visible role models impact on career choices?

Clearly the answers to these questions as well as solutions to the issues in minority pharmacy education requires a multifaceted approach that begins with the individual practitioner. The first steps will be made on this long journey when Hispanic and other minority pharmacists follow their sense of duty to their heritage and their profession to begin promoting and sponsoring their kind in the profession of pharmacy.

## REFERENCES

1. Martin S. Apha House of Delegates to address pharmacists' concerns. Am Pharm 1991;NS31:19-24.

2. Walker PC. Experiential exposure to the pharmacy profession as a minority recruitment tool. Am J Pharm Educ 1988;52:271-6.

3. Hanson EC, Kirk KW. Characteristics of Mexican-American students at one college of pharmacy. Am J Pharm Educ 1987;51:163-5.

4. Weinert AB, Jacoby KE, Gibson RD. Work environment practice attitudes of recent Black and Chicano Doctor of Pharmacy graduates. Am J Pharm Educ 1978;42:295-7.

5. Penna RP, Sherman MS. Degrees conferred by schools and colleges of pharmacy, 1987-1988. Am J Pharm Educ 1989;53:266-83.

6. Westbury I, Purves AC, eds. Cultural literacy and the idea of general education. Chicago: University of Chicago Press, 1988.

7. Poirier S, Lipetz M. Pharmacy in interprofessional education: a course on images of the health professions in the media. Am J Pharm Educ 1987;51:133-7.

8. Henry N, ed. Education for the professions. Chicago: University of Chicago Press, 1962.

9. Albers H. Principles of management: a modern approach. New York: John Wiley & Son, 1974.

10. Carpenito LJ, Duespohl TA. A guide for effective clinical instruction. Wakefield, MA: Nursing Resources, 1981.

# Graduate Pharmaceutical Education: An African-American Perspective

Carolyn M. Brown

**SUMMARY.** This paper reflects my experiences and concerns about graduate education, in particular, from the perspective of an African-American female. As a consequence of being a so-called "double minority" student, I have been provided with various opportunities as well as numerous migraine headaches.

As a minority in a majority institution, I have many unique needs that are generally not satisfied in such institutions. Understanding the concerns of minority students is definitely a prerequisite to providing an atmosphere for higher learning.

In this paper, I will attempt to express some thoughts–in reflections of my needs and concerns–that I think should be considered by institutions who are trying to provide support systems for minority students. In addition, I will offer some suggestions on how to make minorities feel welcome and part of the university system.

I can vividly remember (it was not so long ago!) when I had no idea that I would become a graduate student. Graduate education was the last thing on my mind as I actively pursued my Bachelor's Degree in Pharmacy. Needless to say, at some point, all of that changed. With the encouragement of my professors and the dean at Xavier University of Louisiana, I decided upon pursuing a doctoral degree in Pharmacy Health Care Administration. Thus, it all began.

Upon graduation from pharmacy school in May 1989, I matriculated to the University of Florida to begin my graduate studies. Although I was accepted in other graduate programs, I chose the University of Florida because of its strong commitment to minorities. The University is cur-

---

Carolyn M. Brown, R.Ph., is a graduate student in the Department of Pharmacy Health Care Administration at the University of Florida, P.O. Box 100496, Gainesville, FL 32610.

 

rently doing a good job in providing a support system for minority students. For example, in June 1989, I attended a summer program which was sponsored by the Florida Board of Regents. The purpose of this convocation is to introduce minority students to the joys and rigors of graduate study. It was especially rewarding to me because it enabled me to get acquainted with other African-American students and to get a feel for the University as a whole. This summer program was run by the Office of Graduate Minority Programs.

This office also sponsors visitation programs that provide prospective minority graduate students with information about the University which is relevant in choosing an institution of higher learning. For example, during the visitation program, we were provided with general information about the university such as requirements for admission, housing, expenses, and financial aid. Arrangements were made for us to visit with faculty in our respective areas of interest. In addition, they acquainted us with the social and cultural aspects of the community and furnished us with a basic overview of what living in Gainesville would be like.

I cannot say enough about how much this administration and staff have helped and supported me, both in the past and at present. They have guided me through various problems that I have encountered in connection with the University. For instance, they showed me shortcuts in dealing with the administrative bureaucracy. Furthermore, they have provided me with additional monies such as supplemental fellowships when I was caught in financial binds. In essence, anytime I have had the need for some support, including emotional, social, or financial, there was always someone there to provide that needed support or to guide me in the right direction. As a matter of fact, were it not for these people, I might not be writing this paper today.

The University also houses the Institute of Black Culture which is an educational tool that facilitates Black awareness and enables all races to better understand African Americans and to appreciate their contributions to society. In the presentation of lectures, seminars, forums, tours, and class discussion groups, the institute assists in the joint venture of educating students about the history and cultures of Black peoples the world over.

When I began graduate school in the fall semester of 1989, I was somewhat surprised and perplexed at first. My concerns about and needs for African-American professors had never been more apparent. What I mean is that coming from a Black Catholic university, namely Xavier, I had never really felt the need to have African-American professors because they were always present. However, this was no longer the case.

All of my professors were white males with the exception of three white females in my department. It is sometimes hard for me to be optimistic about obtaining my graduate degree when there is no one around with whom I can fully identify. Even though I strongly feel that I do not lack the scholastic ability to succeed in graduate school, my motivation level occasionally reaches a new all-time low. I have attributed much of this low motivation to the lack of African-Americans in the role of pharmacy educators. Whenever I become overwhelmed with feelings of pessimism, I always turn to my undergraduate professors. They serve as my role models and as living proof that I too can become a professor.

Another situation that I have faced is that, time and time again, I have found myself to be the only African-American student in the classroom. Thanks to Xavier, I have felt neither intimidated nor inferior because of my self-confidence and the feeling of excellence that my alma mater has instilled within me. Nevertheless, I do experience feelings of loneliness. Despite the fact that my fellow students and professors are friendly and respectful, I always lack that feeling of relatedness. It gets especially difficult to learn when you are preoccupied with the fact that there is no one else like you around. It is really important to have other African-American students and professors so that there are people with which we can identify. This will not only benefit African-American students, but it will also enable all students to have a broadened educational experience.

These needs and concerns and feelings of being apart basically constitute my story. I am sure that other minorities have their own story, but I am confident that, at some point, our stories will share common elements. Nevertheless, I have tried to bring out some issues that concern me the most in regards to graduate pharmaceutical education. I have attempted to make known some things that should be considered by majority institutions who are trying to provide support systems for minority students.

First, it must be realized that there are unique forces which operate on African-American people that shape our approach to life. Due to many factors in our cultural background, our thinking styles are different. Second, educators must try to understand our cognitive processes and be able to incorporate this knowledge into their teaching. Third, educators should organize school curricula and programs with the primary purpose of meeting the needs of individual students. I think that this would have the significantly positive effect of providing an atmosphere that is conducive to learning. For instance, during a departmental seminar, I sometimes find myself in a position where I feel the need to "impress" my professors. Needless to say, this kind of unnecessary pressure, whether perceived or real, hinders my ability to perform. In light of such circumstances, those who are trying to support minority education must actively seek to understand the unique needs that shape our being. Finally, until the needs and concerns of minorities are really understood, the problems faced by minorities in majority institutions will never be resolved even on a partial basis. Institutions must make minorities feel welcome and an integral part of the university system.

In closing, I would like to offer a few recommendations to majority institutions who are trying to provide support systems for minority students. First, majority institutions need to actively recruit African-American professors and students. The university should sponsor at least two visitation programs per year that would expose students to what the university has to offer. In addition, universities need to have designated people who will go out to other schools with the expressed purpose of recruiting minority students. However, recruitment is only half of the story and the other half comprises my next suggestion. Recruitment should be followed by plans to retain minority professors and students. Drop out rates have posed an especially serious threat to many efforts to increase enrollment of minority students. One approach to help remedy this situation could be for universities to develop offices of graduate minority programs such as the one at the University of Florida. These offices would serve as sources of support and guidance for minority students. I think that such actions would represent a genuine effort, on the part of the institution, to include minorities as an essential constituent of the university system. Finally, majority institutions should seek to form affiliations with predominantly black universities. This cooperative endeavor could foster a relationship that would enhance the ability to attain a more broadened academic base for all individuals involved. For example, students and faculty from both schools could come together in forums and seminars where thoughts and ideas would be openly exchanged. This would be a learning process for everyone in that they learn from and about each other. In addition, this alliance could make the difficult tasks of both recruiting and retaining African-American professors and students one that can be more easily accomplished. I realize that these suggestions require much time and energy with very careful planning. Nevertheless, any institution that is really interested in providing support systems for minority students will find, in my opinion, that the end result of such hard work was really worth the effort.

In the meantime, however, I am going to continue to pursue a doctoral degree in Pharmacy Health Care Administration for many reasons. However, the primary impetus behind my obtaining a doctoral degree is so that I can serve as a role model to other African-American students. In addition, I am hoping that I can play a part in relieving other African-American students of some of the burdensome problems that I have had to bear.

# Development of Leadership Potential: A Tool for Minorities

Edward H. Clouse

**SUMMARY.** The development of leadership training programs is an essential element in the preparation of nontraditional populations for leadership roles. This article reviews some of the basic characteristics of leadership and the management process of leading and looks at the nature of leadership and the use of power. In addition, the article reviews the early stages of leadership training program development. Also discussed is a progressive leadership development perspective that incorporates personal leadership development, affilial group leadership development, and diverse group leadership development into a program of course work and leadership activities for minorities.

## *INTRODUCTION*

In the business and political world, leadership is probably one of the most talked about, written about, and researched topics in existence.

Edward H. Clouse, Ph.D., is Associate Professor of Pharmacy Administration at Southeastern University of the Health Sciences, 1750 N.E. 168th Street, North Miami Beach, FL 33162. Dr. Clouse is also Executive Director of Phi Lambda Sigma National Pharmacy Leadership Society.

 

Many people seem acutely interested in determining what it takes to be an effective leader in today's complex and changing society. What characteristics does a person need to possess in order to be an effective leader? Why is one leadership style more effective in a given situation than another? In fact, in the field of management, the process of leading is considered one of the four basic functions of proponents of the discipline, along with planning, organizing, and controlling. In this context, leading is considered to encompass all of the following activities: ordering, or indicating what needs to be done; supervising, or being concerned with the training and discipline of subordinates; motivating, or selecting methods that provide subordinates with a reason for executing orders; coordinating, or the act of assembling and synchronizing people and activities so that they interact appropriately in the attainment of objectives; and communicating. This last activity is the primary key to effective leading because, unless a leader can communicate what needs to be done, how it is to be done, by whom it is to be done, and why it is to be done, the success of the entire system can be greatly jeopardized. Leadership, then, is obviously one of those elusive attributes that either allow or prevent certain individuals from obtaining success in their respective positions. Unfortunately, in spite of all this attention to the subject, surprisingly little is known about the leadership process.

Leadership is also a fairly nebulous concept that can mean different things at different times. Most Americans would agree that George Washington, Theodore Roosevelt, and John Kennedy were exemplary leaders. History, however, reveals that Joseph Stalin and Adolf Hitler were equally effective in their own way. In the world of professional sports, several individuals have become noteworthy for taking losing teams and transferring them into winners, and then being fired because of personality clashes with other people within the organization. *Fortune* magazine has also been noted for honoring successful entrepreneurs with vastly different leadership styles. Frederick Crawford, the founder of TRW, was inducted into the Hall of Fame for Business Leadership in 1980, with his success being attributed to his belief in cooperation and communication (1). At the same time, the magazine described the success of Harold Geneen at ITT, who supposedly set unrealistically high goals, expected his managers to obtain them, and publicly humiliated those who failed (2). In spite of the level of study done on leadership, most researchers in the field cannot explain these contradictions and inconsistencies. It is generally agreed, however, that there are certain attributes that can be developed in a person that will enhance leadership potential. This is especially significant for educators of minorities, because minorities have traditionally not assumed, or been permitted to assume, leadership roles.

## *THE NATURE OF LEADERSHIP*

The American Heritage Dictionary defines leadership as the ability to influence others (3). This definition assumes that one understands the related concepts of power, influence, and authority. Power is the ability or capacity to act or perform effectively (3). Influence exists when a person directly or indirectly exercises power to affect a person's behavior or a course of events (3). Authority is power given to a person or a group by an organization (3). Leaders, then, have both power and influence. Depending on their situation, they may not have authority.

According to French and Raven, there are usually five kinds of power found in organizations (4). Legitimate power is power granted through the organizational hierarchy, so the power that occupying a position confers is part of the way that position is defined. Legitimate power is equivalent to authority. Reward power is the power to give or withhold such things as salary increases, bonuses, promotions, praise, recognition, and interesting job assignments. Coercive power is the power to force compliance by use of psychological, emotional or physical threats. Referent power is based on identification, imitation or charisma. In other words, people may react favorably to a leader because they perceive that leader to be like them in personality, background, or attitudes. The fifth kind of power is expert power, which is derived from information or expertise. Obviously, the more important the information and the fewer the people who have access to it, the greater the degree of expert power possessed by any one individual.

It is important for organizations to understand these five kinds of power in order to distinguish between management and leadership. French and Raven claim that management is founded on legitimate, reward, and coercive power. Leadership may also draw on the above powers, but it usually depends more on referent and expert power. In other words, a person may be either a manager or a leader, but not necessarily both. Obviously, from the standpoint of the organization, it is preferable to have managers who are also good leaders. Much of the preoccupation with leadership, then, stems from the fact that organizations want to increase the number of their people who are both managers and leaders. This should be done without preference for race, color, national origin, gender, religion or handicap.

## *LEADERSHIP DEVELOPMENT PROGRAMS*

In recent years, leadership development programs have gained in popularity in response to a need to increase the number and quality of leaders, particularly at the college level. According to Bennett, events in 1984 led to a new level of consciousness in America regarding leadership roles for nontraditional populations (5). The 1984 presidential campaign was historic because a black man was recognized as a major contender for the Democratic presidential nomination and a woman was named the Democratic nominee for vice president. The prominence that these two nontraditional leaders achieved was extremely inspiring to many Americans, especially young women, blacks, and other minorities who felt they possessed the potential to become future leaders in American society.

The concept of developing student leadership at the college level through education and systematic training programs had already been supported by several educators around the country (6-8). According to Young, adopting such procedures for the development of nontraditional populations should increase the pool of leadership talent by 1) identifying members of nontraditional populations as potential leaders 2) educating them to acquire knowledge of basic leadership principles, and 3) providing training opportunities for them to learn skills and behaviors for leadership roles and services on diverse levels, including personal, family, campus organizations, community organizations, careers, and public services (9). The purpose of the leadership development programs, then, is to bring more minorities into the mainstream of American society and its political, economic, and educational institutions (10). This can be done through education and systematic training programs with special attention focused on providing appropriate leadership experiences for nontraditional student populations.

Guthrie and Miller recommend augmenting courses and activities with three progressive leadership development perspectives that focus specifically on some of the perceived leadership development needs of nontraditional populations (7). These three perspectives are personal leadership development, affilial group leadership development, and diverse group leadership development.

Personal leadership development involves self-awareness, self-growth, and self-actualization. Self-awareness is encouraged through assessment of one's personality, including beliefs, needs, values, philosophies, interests, strengths, weaknesses, and goals. Growth is encouraged through self-discipline, management and resolution of inner conflict, plans to achieve goals, holistic health efforts, and multifaceted involvement and service. Actual growth can then be measured by goal attainment, contributions, self-esteem, and a sense of personal fulfillment. Success in this area of leadership development should prepare the participants for advancement to the next level. It is up to the instructor to decide when advancement should occur.

Affilial group leadership development involves affilial group identification, affilial group esteem, and affilial group unity and support. Identification is encouraged through awareness of the affilial group, acknowledgment of one's membership within the group, knowledge of personal and group homogeneity, communication, involvement and mentorship regarding group needs, concerns, and goals. Esteem is developed through confidence generated from active service. Such service is also useful in promoting affilial group pride, unity, and support, all important qualities to a nontraditional leader. As before, mastery of this area of leadership development should prepare the participants for further advancement.

Diverse group leadership development involves awareness and recognition of diverse groups, sensitivity and respect for diverse groups, and mutuality with diverse groups. Awareness and recognition are encouraged through knowledge of diverse group's heterogeneity. Sensitivity and respect are promoted through active involvement with diverse groups, open communication in planning, implementing, and evaluating shared efforts, conflict resolution, and concern for the human rights of diverse groups. Mutuality is encouraged through recognition of shared goals and realization of common interests and interdependence in attaining goals set for the mutual benefit of diverse groups.

## *CONCLUSION*

Although leadership has been studied in great detail, very little is known about the process. Most organizations prefer to employ people who are leaders as well as managers. In order to prepare leaders for the future, education and systematic training programs are needed. Educational institutions can help meet this need through courses, activities, and programs in leadership development. Particular attention must be given to developing leadership potential in nontraditional populations, such as women, blacks, and other minorities. One method discussed for accomplishing this involves augmenting courses and activities with personal leadership development, affilial group leadership development, and diverse group leadership development. These three progressive leadership development perspectives focus specifically on some of the perceived leadership development needs of nontraditional populations. These perspectives are intended to be mastered individually and progression is determined by the respective instructor.

One element not discussed in this article is that of recognition. Recognition of leadership potential can be an essential tool in the continued development of an individual's capabilities. In the profession of pharmacy, this need has been addressed since 1965 by an organization created primarily for students. The purpose of Phi Lambda Sigma, the National Pharmacy Leadership Society, is to promote the development of leadership qualities, especially among pharmacy students. By peer recognition, the Society encourages participation in all pharmacy activities. Since membership crosses fraternal and organizational lines, the Society does not compete with any other organization. No greater honor can be bestowed upon a person than to be recognized as a leader by peers. Such recognition serves to instill self-confidence and to promote greater efforts toward the advancement of pharmacy. Furthermore, peer recognition encourages the less active student to assume a more active role.

## REFERENCES

1. Holt DD. The hall of fame for business leadership. Fortune 1980;(Apr 21):101-9.

2. Menzies HD. The ten toughest bosses. Fortune 1980;(Apr 21):62-73.

3. Boyer M et al. The American heritage dictionary. New York: Dell Publishing Co., Inc., 1986.

4. French J, Raven B. The bases of social power. Studies in social power. Ann Arbor, MI: University of Michigan Press, 1959:150-67.

5. Bennett L. Black politics: the road to freedom? Ebony 1984;34(Aug):34-6.

6. Hyman RT. Improving discussion leadership. New York: Columbia University, Teachers College Press, 1980.

7. Guthrie E, Miller WS. Process politics: a guide for group leaders. San Diego, CA: University Associates, 1981.

8. Lassey WR, Sashkin M. Leadership and social change. San Diego, CA: University Associates, 1983.

9. Young JL. Developing nontraditional leaders. J Multicultural Counsel Develop 1986;7(July):108-15.

10. Willie CV. Leadership development programs for minorities: an evaluation. Urban Rev 1984;16(Apr):209-17.

# The Mexican American Association of Pharmacy Students (MAAPS)

Leticia de la Rosa

**SUMMARY.** The Mexican American Association of Pharmacy Students (MAAPS) was organized at the University of Texas at Austin by a group of Hispanics of Mexican descent who shared common professional interests, values and cultural backgrounds. The members of this organization perform many activities for the College of Pharmacy including: assisting in recruiting, retaining qualified students who have been accepted into pharmacy school, providing health care education to the community and maintaining open communication channels between the students and the College administration.

The members benefit from the support they receive from each other and through their involvement in various service projects. Their activities make a difference in the community. One of the most important examples of these is "Project Mentorship." The objective here is to assist in the development and retention of minority children in elementary school, especially those at high risk of failure. Mentors must devote at least thirty (30) minutes per week in order to participate.

Students, the College of Pharmacy and the community all benefit from MAAPS involvement and activity. This is a good example of how social and professional networks help in minority pharmaceutical education.

The Mexican American Association of Pharmacy Students (MAAPS) became a recognized campus organization in fall 1981. It was organized by a group of Mexican Americans who shared common professional interests, values and cultural backgrounds.

Despite the fact that the organization was brought into existence by a group of Mexican-American students, the members represent a variety of

---

Leticia de la Rosa is President of MAAPS and a pharmacy student at the University of Texas at Austin College of Pharmacy, Austin, TX 78712.

 

cultures and backgrounds. MAAPS encourages all qualified students to join. A small percentage of the members are prepharmacy students. These students enjoy the contact with others already in the college. The close rapport they develop increases their confidence in reaching their goals in pharmacy.

The organization has accomplished many objectives since its beginning: assisting in recruitment; retaining qualified students within the College of Pharmacy; providing health care education to the community; and maintaining open communication channels between students and the College administration. These objectives have been met by the members through sponsoring drug awareness programs and conducting hypertension and diabetic screening services for the Mexican-American community of East Austin.

The members benefit from this organization through the friends they make and through their involvement in service activities that make a difference in the community. After all, our profession is exactly that, one of caring.

## *PROJECT MENTORSHIP*

One of our most recent service projects is called "Mentorship." It is organized in conjunction with the Austin Independent School District. The objective of this project is to assist in the development and retention of minority children in school. The children with which we work are considered high risk, more likely to fall into destructive life-styles, such as alcohol or drug abuse. They are identified by their teachers and are referred to the principal or campus coordinator for the project. A MAAPS mentor is then assigned to work with the child who has similar interests and hobbies.

Each mentor is asked to devote at least thirty minutes each week to this project. If the they can afford more time to see the child more often, they are encouraged to do so. Although the children are excused from class when the mentor visits, the mentor is asked to come when it is mutually convenient. It is apparent that this program is very important to the schools. The teachers have expressed great enthusiasm when we visit and have even shared stories with us of students who have already shown improvement in just the two months since the program's inception. The parents, particularly the mothers, have also shown great interest and encourage the participation of their children.

When a mentor visits a child, it is a special time that they share together. They may go to the library to read a book or take a walk together around the campus to share thoughts. In the beginning, the child is often shy and inhibited, but with time the barriers fall away and they become comfortable with each other allowing a special trust and friendship to be formed.

The members in our organization have been alerted to the problems of our Hispanic population. By assisting in these types of projects, they are brought to the core of the problem. We become involved and then, can understand better the needs of the Hispanic disadvantaged children. Thirty minutes a week is so little time that you might think it could not make a difference. But just the opposite is true. The children eagerly await their mentor's arrival, ready to show off good grades, to tell stories and to demonstrate how good they feel to have a special friend. The members who participate in this service project are rewarded time and time again by the reports of good conduct, improved attendance and scholastic achievement. We are making a difference.

Keeping these children interested in education also does a world of good for the community. With the difference that we are making, there is a good chance many of these children will not fall victim to the same problems as other high risk students who do not have the safety net of the Mentorship Program. Many community problems seem to stem from teenagers who have dropped out of school. These drop-outs tend to live a life of crime and drug abuse and become a burden to society. The children participating in this program often have a sibling or parent who is involved in some kind of destructive life-style. It is often difficult to compete with these familial role models, but if we can keep their interest focused on education we are on the right track toward improving our community.

## *OTHER PROJECTS*

In the 1989 fall semester, MAAPS became affiliated with the South Austin Youth Services (SAYS). This organization is a federally funded outreach program that assists underprivileged and at-risk Hispanic and Black families and young people in this area. MAAPS and SAYS joined forces to motivate students to stay in school and to inform them about career opportunities in pharmacy. As the semester progressed, we participated in their family health festival, gave tours of the pharmacy school to at-risk teens, donated funds to their Thanksgiving Dinner and hosted speakers to learn more about outreach programs. We continue to be a resource for SAYS in providing guidance and support to the disadvantaged Hispanic youth in South Austin.

Another important service project in which MAAPS members look forward to participating every spring is the Vial of Life Program. We distribute plastic vials to the parts of Austin that are predominantly Hispanic. Each contains a form on which a person can write important medical information (e.g., present medical condition, allergies, current medication). The vial is then attached to a rack in the person's refrigerator, then a decal indicating program participation is placed on the person's front door. When needed, Emergency Medical Services personnel have been trained to look for the vial. This process can save precious time and supply valuable information. MAAPS members really enjoy participating in this service project. It gives us an opportunity to practice our communication skills and, at the same time, serve the community. One woman actually called us to say that the Vial of Life Program saved her husband's life and to express how very grateful she was.

Each fall, MAAPS members dress up in their favorite costumes and attend the Travis State School Halloween party to serve as assistants to staff. The majority of the clients here are mentally retarded or suffer from multiple sclerosis. The work load is divided into four shifts of forty-five minutes each, though we usually volunteer for the entire evening. The clients are brought to us and we escort them around the gymnasium to various games and food booths. If a client lacks the necessary motor skills to feed himself, it is our responsibility to assist him. The school provides corn dogs and hot dogs as well as a variety of games such as the ring toss, basketball throw and horseshoes. In addition, there are several haunted houses. While the supplies are all furnished, MAAPS members provide smiles and companionship for the evening. This service project is very rewarding for our members. Not only does it make us appreciate all the blessings we enjoy, but it also makes us more patient and understanding of the needs of others.

Another service project in which MAAPS members participate is blood pressure screening. Members are trained by the professional personnel at the University of Texas Student Health Center. They learn the importance of maintaining normal blood pressure and how to use a sphygmomanometer. We distribute literature from the American Heart Association on the causes of hypertension and on proper nutrition. If a pressure is screened above normal, the patient is advised to seek further medical attention.

As you can see our members keep very busy.

# The Advantages of a Minority Attending Historically Black Colleges and Universities

Marilyn D. Saulsbury

**SUMMARY.** There are many reasons for Black students to attend Historically Black Colleges and Universities (HBCUs). The low student-to-teacher ratio is a definitive factor for many Black students, in which the possibility of requesting and getting individual help, if necessary, is achievable. Secondly, a feeling of unified competitiveness to succeed not only individually, but as a race, is a positive factor.

Moreover, young Black students are welcomed on the basis of their academic, social or artistic talents, with no reference to fulfilling a racial quota. Furthermore, at HBCUs, Black students have role models who perpetuate the belief that all people have the right and capability to learn and excel in all fields of study. Finally, Black students feel a renewed sense of pride in themselves when they attend Black institutions of higher learning.

There are many advantages for minorities at Historically Black Colleges and Universities. This article will summarize many of the factors that are important to the writer and which were determinants for her choosing a predominantly Black university in order to study pharmacy.

One of the most important factors for non-Whites going to a historically black institution of higher learning is the low ratio of students to teacher. The small class sizes enhance the interaction between pupils and faculty. We are able to go to a professor at any time to ask questions about classes or career choices. S/He is not just a student who possesses a Social Security Card and no face, they are unique individuals with

Marilyn D. Saulsbury is a pharmacy student at Xavier University of Louisiana College of Pharmacy, New Orleans, LA 70125.

 

special talents and needs. In this way, the Black student benefits having not only an instructor, but also an advisor who cares.

Furthermore, competitiveness is viewed differently at Black universities than at majority institutions. Non-Black students at non-Black schools compete against each other with temerity and cut-throat ferocity. In this environment, some students will flourish and some will not, but overall, due to the large number of non-Black students, more will have the opportunity to complete school, get jobs and live a nice life with hard work and sacrifice. At Black institutions, even though competition is good, if you lose a student, you lose a potentially hard-working Black American who can contribute to the continued efforts to help his/her race.

Because being a minority means being small in number compared to the majority, Blacks cannot afford to lose even one individual if we wish to continue to combat the adversities of everyday life as Black Americans. For this reason, students who are excelling academically and teachers at Black institutions, generally cannot afford the luxury of basking in praise or resting on their laurels, because they feel motivated to help their brothers and sisters who are not succeeding as well. This idea of sacrificing to help others helps the motivated student and the local and national Black community.

Black students who attend Black schools also receive a feeling of belonging and welcome. They know that they will be accepted for their academic, social or artistic talents, with no reference to race. A feeling of acceptance for any individual is important. When a person feels accepted and wanted, they actively produce and complete tasks given to them. Also, if they are really motivated and impressed by those around them, they attempt to emulate what is seen and felt. Thus, going to Black institutions with other Black students and with professors who accept them and expect them to do well, offers positive reinforcement. This fosters role models who will continue this experience to other Black students of the future. When one is surrounded by positive role models, the morale and expectations of the individual reflects one's environment. Black institutions perpetuate the belief that all people have the innate right to learn and excel in fields of study that interest them.

Ninety percent (90%) of all Black professionals in America graduated from Historically Black Colleges or Universities. Attending a Black institution of higher learning prepares students to meet the challenges they will face daily. Graduates leave with confidence, self-worth, determination and a fervent desire to beat the odds. This urgency to prove their competence as trained and skilled professionals has a triad effect.

Initially, Black students have a compelling drive to succeed for their families/guardians or ancestors who have come before them. Even though many Black students have immediate or distant family who have graduated from college, a great number of them have no relatives who have attended an institution of higher learning. For this reason, they become the first person to complete college. With these types of expectations from their parents and other relatives resting upon their shoulders, Black students strive to do well. They owe a debt to their family who helped them financially. Moreover, they feel a deep emotional and psychological commitment to excel, because when they do, their entire family excels.

Secondly, the Black student has to prove to herself that she can utilize her knowledge and talents to achieve the "American Dream." A disproportionate number of minority students do not possess the financial and social advantages of nonminority students. Thus, many Black students are not able to experience a variety of cultural and social enlightenings of their non-Black schoolmates. The ability to go to dramatic plays, operas, ballet, symphony concerts, museums, galleries, school debates and scholastic competitions is not possessed by all Black students. Additionally, for those Black students who may be financially or academically able to afford participation in these activities, the time factor is important. Managing time between school and working to cover expenses is difficult and leaves little chance for cultural outings. Yet, Black-student graduates want to be able to afford and enjoy the finer things in life, rather than just get by.

Finally, Black students wish to prove continuously to non-Blacks that they are intelligent and resourceful people who are able to perform at any job or task that they are given. They also want to show that they are worthy of their jobs, not because they are Black and maintain a quota for the workplace, but because they worked hard for their position and can produce as workers or managers.

Along with fulfilling these dreams, young Black Americans learn the extreme importance of supporting Black schools which help support Black people. They demonstrate this by giving back to Black institutions financially. This helps to continue the upkeep and maintenance of historically Black schools. Moreover, Black alumni can encourage and send their children or relatives to attend these institutions which foster the continuation of their important presence in Black America.

## *CONCLUSION*

There are many reasons for Black students to attend Historically Black Colleges and Universities. The first is the low student to teacher ratio.

This number is such that each student is able to have personal interactions with his/her instructors. This is most helpful for students to get assistance with their course work and to ask questions about tentative careers.

Second is the feeling of unified competitiveness that is present at Black institutions. Here, Black students and professors help not only themselves but others in the Black community who may not have the opportunity to have a better life-style.

Thirdly, young Black students receive a feeling of belonging and being welcomed for themselves. This helps them to succeed without reference to their skin color and other prejudicial stereotypes.

Additionally, at predominately Black institutions, Black students have an abundance of Black role models who help perpetuate the belief that all people have the right to learn and excel in fields of study that are of interest to them.

Finally, when Black students attend Black universities, they gain a renewed pride in the accomplishments of their peers. They also become confident and determined to prove to non-Blacks that they are worthy of their achievements, not as a quota or a number, but because of their individual abilities.

# Understanding Minority Education in Pharmacy

Barry Bleidt

At Xavier University, we have a saying, "there is no such thing as problems, only opportunities."

**SUMMARY.** Minority education is an economic, societal and altruistic issue. One out of every three wage earners, by the year 2000, will be minorities. If a large percentage of these individuals are not economically empowered, societal productivity and social security, among other things, will suffer greatly. Pharmacy offers an excellent opportunity for economic advancement.

The key to success in muticultural pharmaceutical education is commitment–long-term, unwavering commitment. Historically Black Colleges and Universities have shown this strategy to be most effective. Majority institutions need to emulate some of their tactics in order to succeed.

Different types of support groups are needed by students in order to increase their chances for success. Academic, professional and social networks are each very important ingredients. Also, cultural sensitivity toward all students is paramount. It makes the individual feel and act important.

Ethnic diversity is healthy and good. Striving to achieve it is not easy, but well worth the effort. Using many of the suggestions from the entire special volume, institutions desiring to endeavor into this meaningful and rewarding activity (i.e., increasing the number of minority pharmacists) can and will succeed. Early science-education pipelines, the Carolyn Brown effect and the nature of commitment are but some of the advice offered.

Read well, take notes, call for additional information and try, by all means, try–all students and the profession will benefit.

The purpose of this special edition devoted to "Multicultural Pharmaceutical Education" was to bring the spotlight better into focus on an

---

Barry Bleidt, Ph.D., is Associate Professor of Pharmacy Administration at the Xavier University of Louisiana College of Pharmacy, New Orleans, LA 70125.

 

important topic and to present a collection of ideas on what minority education is about. In this, we have succeeded. Thirteen articles have discussed various aspects of the subject. Commitment, concern and courage have been addressed.

For the attuned reader, this compilation has provided valuable suggestions on how to increase the chances of success in improving a track record of attracting and retaining minority students. Others have gleaned information that will benefit their institution in establishing a long-term goal of expanding the pool of minority pharmacists or postbaccalaureate graduates. Many barriers have been detailed along with the means to overcome them.

## *INTRODUCTION*

The societal marketplace in the United States will be different in the future not only for higher education, but also for goods and services. Minorities will soon make up the majority. The impact of this phenomena will be awe inspiring and potentially devastating, especially if actions are not taken now anticipating these changes.

The low availability of skilled workers already threatens some industries and our international competitive posture. More groups are pursuing smaller numbers of potential students and employees. Pharmacy schools must compete with engineering and other health professional programs as well as environmental and biotechnology interests. The pool of qualified applicants is dwindling in some areas. It has already been predicted that before the turn of the century 45 percent of all students will be classified as nontraditional (older, part-time, etc.). Colleges of pharmacy are already being affected by these changes. Failing to recognize these and plan for the future is planning to fail.

The renewed interest in minority issues as they relate to pharmaceutical education is, in a few cases, genuine altruism for the plight of the disenfranchised. However, for the most part, this concern is brought about by legislative or public pressures and by the need to expand the availability of potential students. While not as socially redeeming as the first reason, the second motivation is real and valid, and can be mutually beneficial to both the institution and minority students if handled properly.

Still others are preparing for the future. One such example is Eli Lilly and Company. Their commitment to minority education and employment is unsurpassed and is an excellent beacon for others to follow. They are dedicated to creating an ethnically diverse work place. Why? First of all, it makes good business sense. The markets of tomorrow require a knowledge of what minorities will need and what will motivate them to buy (who better to provide this information than members of these groups from within the company). Secondly, in order to attract the needed, skilled workers of tomorrow, a company must position itself now. If significant numbers of minorities are already in mid-to upper-level management positions, the company will have improved greatly its marketability to other members of these groups. This, of course, entails hiring and developing employees now. Lilly is doing this and should be greatly commended for their foresight and understanding of the benefits that ethnic diversity brings.

The educationally disadvantaged represent another pool from which pharmacy can draw. This term does not mean that a student is African-American or Hispanic. It indicates that a student comes from a background where the school system's standards are below that which is needed to prepare them adequately for higher education. One such example is found in the Orleans Parish School System where test tubes for chemistry classes (in the very few places that offer them) are considered luxuries. Contrast this to a school that has microscopes, fully furnished science laboratories and good libraries and you can see how some students are disadvantaged long before they reach college. Unfortunately, the largest percentage of these students are minority students from poor inner cities or rural areas. The educational pipeline concept discussed earlier and also later is one way to help combat this problem.

In the following pages, I will be discussing some of the things that this special volume brought to light, the importance of support groups, the Carolyn Brown Effect and cultural sensitivity and access issues as they relate to higher education. In addition, some concluding remarks and acknowledgments will be made.

## *IN THE SPOTLIGHT*

Several significant things were discovered in the course of constructing this special volume. These include the importance of commitment, the role of minority institutions, the function of leadership and the ability of some schools to maintain ethnic diversity with little or no extra effort.

First is the vital part played by commitment. Long-term devotion to minority education is needed in order to succeed. This is why the minority institutions achieve their goals and have their students prosper as a result–COMMITMENT. Dr. Gibson's treatise of the subject is both moving and compelling. Commitment is also why in the 1990s, more minority students, as well as majority ones, are selecting minority institutions to study pharmacy. Majority institutions must now make some major changes in order to compete and expand their applicant pool. The modifications from the upper echelons down must be in the form of a long-term commitment to minority issues. This is the starting point–commitment; without it all attempts will be futile.

Second, the importance of Historically Black Colleges and Universities (HBCUs) in terms of producing pharmacists has been delineated. HBCUs differ from predominately African-American institutions in that they were founded for the special purpose of educating African Americans rather than just having enrollments exceeding 50 percent African-American students (1). Out of the 105 HBCUs, only four have colleges of pharmacy. Without these institutions, the low numbers of practicing African-American pharmacists would be even more abysmally small.

These institutions and their graduates have been the impetus for many of the gains African Americans have achieved, especially between 1960 and 1980. Additionally, their tradition of academic experimentation and teaching methods have provided examples that majority institutions could emulate, not just for minorities, but for all students. Ironically, now questions are being raised about whether or not the African-American colleges are still needed (1). For the sake of the profession, let us hope they do stay around or pharmacy will be even more ethnocentric than it already is.

Third, the function of leadership in minority education among students and institutions was revealed. Role models (abstract ones of like characteristics and familiar ones), leadership training and professional associations are useful tools in developing students for future practice.

Equally important is the recognition of leadership. Without acknowledgment, many individuals cease such positive behaviors. In order to maintain motivation, some official expression of awareness is necessary. Phi Lambda Sigma, the National Pharmacy Leadership Society, is an excellent vehicle to accomplish this purpose. Each school should have a chapter, not just to reward the minority leaders, but to provide something meaningful and prestigious for which all students can strive to achieve.

Fourth, a few universities enjoy an ethnic and/or racial diversity among their students without an organized effort to recruit, retain or assist them specifically. The University of Texas at Austin and Southeastern University of the Health Sciences are two such examples. Certainly, local demographics are in their favor, but this is true of other institutions with low numbers of minorities. What do they do that is so different?

First and foremost, each has a history (even though Southeastern's is relatively new in pharmacy) of providing for their student's needs–something that is required when dealing with minorities.

## *SUPPORT GROUPS*

Majority students at majority universities take many things for granted, as does the administration and the faculty. There are a multitude of forces that contribute to a student's success in a scholastic environment. One of the major keys is the presence of support groups. These networks are vital components to a professional education.

In pharmaceutical education, there are three identifiable support groups that are important in providing the proper atmosphere for achievement. They are not necessarily mutually exclusive, nor are they generally the same. These are the academic, social and professional networks. Each is uniquely important in shaping the practicing pharmacist of tomorrow.

Most schools recognize the importance of the academic support group in both majority and minority education and exert some effort toward retaining those already admitted into professional programs. Rho Chi tutors, mentoring, recorded lectures and study groups are but a few of the means utilized to assist students scholastically. Extra undertakings also are employed sometimes to ensure that minority students are given additional chances of succeeding.

While these tactics are helpful (in many cases), attention should also be focused on providing support in the other two areas. The social network for all students is crucial to their development and mental well-being. At a majority institution, this support group is generally taken for granted, especially by majority students and faculty. But to the minority student, its absence can present a significant barrier. Attention should be paid to this detail. One successful example was presented in Carolyn Brown's article: the University of Florida supports and maintains an Institute of Black Culture, the purpose of which is to act as "an educational tool that facilitates Black awareness and enables all races to better understand African Americans and to appreciate their contribution to society." Another example was cited in Marilyn Saulsbury's paper on the advantages of minorities attending Historically Black Colleges and Universities.

It is insufficient to assume that minority students will seek out each other and build a network. The successful university (at least in terms of recruiting and keeping minorities) will be proactive in ensuring that the social needs of these students are met. Cultural activities, red-tape reduction, special programs are a few of the methods that work. Minorities are individuals and have distinctive differences among them and to think otherwise is cultural insensitivity (or worse).

The last type of support group is the professional one. Preceptors, teachers, professional society members and role models are among the contacts that enable students to flourish. In a health care profession such as pharmacy, this network is equally important to the others. Within it, students mature and develop connections for future employment and such. The Student National Pharmaceutical Association (SNPhA) and the Mexican American Association of Pharmacy Students (at U.T. Austin) are two prime examples of this network in action.

Professionalism is best developed by emulating how other pharmacists act or perform. Regular communication with others provides the opportunity to acquire this needed proficiency. Once a school has sufficient numbers, establishing a SNPhA chapter is a vital tool in supporting a professional network for African-American pharmacy students and others.

Universities aspiring to succeed in attracting and retaining minorities should pay attention to the details necessary to accomplish their goals. Understanding and providing the proper support groups are two such components in this equation. A proactive approach with caring and sensitivity works and comes highly recommended.

## *CAROLYN BROWN EFFECT*

During the past decade of academic service, I have attended a myriad of seminars on the virtues of graduate education after pharmacy school. Most were informative, some interesting, but none very motivating in terms of its effect on the intended audience. Recently, as part of my pharmacy management class, I invited a Xavierite, now a graduate student at the University of Florida, to speak to the group about her experiences in quaternary education.

Carolyn Brown was a recent graduate (less than twenty months) from the College of Pharmacy. The impact of her talk was tremendous. The students' responses were overwhelmingly positive. No less than six members (fifteen percent) of the class have applied to a graduate program, many as a result of Ms. Brown's presentation.

Was it because Ms. Brown was so dynamic or gave information heretofore unpresented? Not really. Was it because she was an African-American female role model that drove the point home? Partly, however, the

Carolyn Brown Effect is the fact that many of the students knew her personally and remembered her from school.

The students actually could identify with Carolyn on a personal basis. This was especially true when she made the point about sitting where they were (usually bored !!) two years ago and now she was nearly half way finished with her doctorate. The general feeling among the students was, "I could do that." Many are going to try. The impact was incredible and immediate.

Once an institution is able to recruit one or two students from an area where large numbers of minority students live, employing the "Carolyn Brown Effect" will attract more. This has two benefits. One, to the institution, in terms of increasing the ethnic diversity of the student body. And two, to the student, it provides an opportunity to go home and say, "Look, I've made it and so can you" and maybe earn additional income as a recruiter (if they are lucky).

This technique will work at both the graduate level and undergraduate level (especially, if you use first-year students or ones recently accepted into pharmacy school). Of course, the first step is to bring on board those crucial first ones to set the stage for those who will follow.

## *CREATE AN EDUCATIONAL PIPELINE*

One way to attract the first minorities to your institution is to create an educational pipeline. As part of the long-term strategy, develop programs that will strengthen the science and mathematics background of disadvantaged or high-risk students, thereby lowering their riskiness. Not only will such programs accomplish the educational goals, they also will demonstrate that your school has a caring attitude and is trying to meet the needs of minority communities–an important image to have.

The many, many years of success that Xavier University of Louisiana has enjoyed in preparing African Americans for pharmacy and other sciences is *NOT* only because it is a historically Black institution. In the article by Dr. J. W. Carmichael et al., the evolution of a series of programs designed to reach students earlier in their education is discussed and its effect chronicled.

I do believe, however, that the reason such innovative programs were initiated was because Xavier is committed to furthering the higher educational aspirations of African Americans. XU's mission also permitted the flexibility needed to experiment in order to discover what works for the traditionally disenfranchised. Readers should take advantage of the knowledge gained through the educational research conducted at HBCUs.

The pipeline concept entails intervening just as many students begin to drop out (eighth grade). Analytical-reasoning skills, mathematics and science programs are needed by many coming from educationally-disadvantaged backgrounds. Summer sessions, social events and school visitation activities along with concerned faculty and staff are elements of a successful pipeline that will assist in developing your students of tomorrow. Go back and read the article by Dr. Carmichael et al. carefully. It provides the details of how the system works.

## *CULTURAL SENSITIVITY*

Another key factor is understanding: understanding the differences among cultures, among religions, among individuals. This compassion is known as cultural sensitivity. Just having an awareness of ethno-specific distinctions is insufficient. An institution must exude a caring feeling towards those who are minority in order to make them feel comfortable and augment their chances of success, thereby increasing the desirability (to them) of attending your school.

Figure 1 presents the evolutionary steps from cultural insensitivity to cultural integration. One of the obstacles in this process is moving from cultural awareness to cultural sensitivity. For some reason, it is much easier to be aware of the ethno-specific dissimilarities and to appreciate the art, music and other cultural heritages of minorities than it is to accept them as equals and treat them accordingly.

Cultural sensitivity in higher education involves the following factors:

1. recognizing and understanding ethno-specific problems (such as racism or anti-Semitism);
2. respecting the person as a human being and their rights to be treated as one;
3. communicating in a cross-cultural fashion at the student's (consumer's) level, especially in learning situations without being condescending;
4. being a good listener, being empathetic and being *polite*;
5. understanding, without judgment, differing value systems and beliefs that the student may hold;
6. linking with the disenfranchised, using alternative or counter-cultural contacts or techniques, if necessary;
7. identifying from where the person comes–poverty, religion, little

formal schooling, language, cultural heritage–and using this to link with them;
8. accepting those who may be different as equals;
9. using innovative approaches from other cultures to solve individual problems (the student's, the institution's and other's);
10. demonstrating a *genuine* concern for their well-being and, where applicable, the student's homeland;
11. sharing a part of yourself with the student;
12. learning constantly about other cultures; and
13. appreciating the differences among cultures.

Another concern is one about access to higher education. Many students face hurdles along their way to matriculating. These obstructions must be dealt with whenever discussing minority issues. While nearly 50 percent of African Americans and many Hispanic Americans are middle class or above economically, the vast majority of those who live in poverty or are near poor (125% of poverty level) belong to these two groups.

In addition to the lack of financial wherewithal, other barriers to access include:

- lack of knowledge about available loans, grants and programs;
- educationally disadvantaged backgrounds;
- culturally insensitive institutions;
- cultural beliefs toward pharmacy or education, in general;
- previous, unpleasant experiences;
- lack of role models;
- transportation;
- inaccessible building or facilities (for people with disablities);
- out of a service area (no program nearby);
- lack of affordable places to live;
- disenfranchised, not part of mainstream society; and
- individual student motivation.

| CULTURAL INSENSITIVITY (Ethnocentricity) | ⇨ | CULTURAL AWARENESS | ⇨ | CULTURAL SENSITIVITY | ⇨ | CULTURAL INTEGRATION (Ethnic Diversity) |
|---|---|---|---|---|---|---|

FIGURE 1. The evolution towards cultural integration within society.

## *CONCLUSION*

First, I would like to acknowledge the hard work put forth by each contributor. Their concern demonstrates what it takes to be successful in minority education–commitment. The author's efforts are greatly appreciated. It is now up to the readers to make their activities pay off.

It is not that minority education is so different from a good majority education that is the point; there are few, if any, dissimilarities. However, an understanding of history, culture, individual backgrounds and other tangential issues is needed in order to focus on providing opportunities to succeed.

In order to prosper in multicultural pharmaceutical education, an institution needs to do three things–*COMMIT*, *COMMIT*, and *COMMIT*. With these, everything else works itself out.

One of the key messages that should be received from this special volume is that a move toward improving an institution's situation must be considered a long-term project with the idea of getting long-term results. In the short run, outcomes will hardly be measurable, if at all. The articles from Florida A&M University and Ohio State University and by Dr. Carmichael et al. demonstrate the advantages of adopting this type of philosophy.

The primary reason, I believe, for many failures in this area has been insufficient follow-through. Five, ten, even fifteen years are considered short term for these types of societal changes. Too often, it occurs that a project to improve the status of minorities in pharmacy is terminated in favor of other competing priorities with less overall societal benefit and significance.

Another point that I would like to make is on the definition of a high-risk student. Dr. Montagne's article on advantaging the disadvantaged student pokes holes in the standard definition of chancy admittees. As he points out, far too often, criteria are utilized to place a person into the inadmissible category based on improper discrimination. It is time to revisit our definitions, not lower standards, and find ways to include the disenfranchised within pharmacy education. The traditional, full-time over-five-year student is disappearing. Six-year programs and less-than-full-time students are becoming the norm. What real difference does it make to society whether a student finishes their entry-level degree in six, seven, eight or more years?

Ethnic diversity is good for almost any institution. It provides different points of view on events and problems that can lead to better solutions. In a business sense, cultural variety opens new markets and expands existing ones. Institutions of higher learning need to think more in this vein, rather than remain in the old ivory tower where the view is generally clouded.

The solution, of course, is really very simple: consider the individual differences in us all as worthy of recognition and respect each of us as human beings.

## REFERENCE

1. Garibaldi A, ed. Black colleges: an overview. Black colleges and universities. New York: Praeger Publishers, 1984.

* 9 7 8 0 7 8 9 0 0 0 7 1 2 *
T - #0568 - 101024 - C0 - 212/152/9 - PB - 9780789000712 - Gloss Lamination